Preparing for the Physical Therapist
Licensure Examination

Patricia Rae Evans, MEd, PT
Associate Professor and Chair
Department of Health and Human Sciences
Samuel Merritt College
Oakland, California

F. A. DAVIS COMPANY • Philadelphia

F. A. Davis Company
1915 Arch Street
Philadelphia, PA 19103

Printed in the United States of America

Last digit indicates print number: 10 9 8 7 6 5 4 3 2 1

Publisher, Health Professions: Jean-François Vilain
Developmental Editor: Christa Fratantoro
Production Editor: Stephen D. Johnson
Cover Designer: Louis J. Forgione

As new scientific information becomes available through basic and clinical research, recommended treatments and drug therapies undergo changes. The author and publisher have done everything possible to make this book accurate, up to date, and in accord with accepted standards at the time of publication. The author, editors, and publisher are not responsible for errors or omissions or for consequences from application of the book, and make no warranty, expressed or implied, in regard to the contents of the book. Any practice described in this book should be applied by the reader in accordance with professional standards of care used in regard to the unique circumstances that may apply in each situation. The reader is advised always to check product information (package inserts) for changes and new information regarding dose and contraindications before administering any drug. Caution is especially urged when using new or infrequently ordered drugs.

Library of Congress Cataloging-in-Publication Data

Evans, Patricia Rae, 1939–
    Preparing for the physical therapist licensure examination /
Patricia Rae Evans.
        p.   cm.
    Includes bibliographical references.
    ISBN 0-8036-0251-0 (alk. paper)
    1. Physical therapy Examinations, questions, etc.   I. Title.
    [DNLM: 1. Physical Therapy Examination Questions.   WB 18.2 E92p
1999]
RM701.6.E94 1999
615.8′2′076—dc21
DNLM/DLC
for Library of Congress   99-22839
                                                                         CIP

I would like to dedicate this book to my mother, Oolah, for always believing in me and for teaching me to have a servant's heart.

This book provides the reader with a comprehensive overview of the requirements to enter physical therapy practice at the close of the 20th century. The review book has been developed for physical therapists, educated in the United States and abroad, who are preparing to take the licensure examination. It is specifically designed to correspond with the content outlines developed by the Federation of State Boards of Physical Therapy in 1997 following its extensive analysis of physical therapy practice.

Chapter 1 provides a thorough description of the examination itself and offers suggestions for organizing your preparation as well as test-taking techniques. Chapters 2, 3, and 4 provide, respectively, the three areas of the content outlines—assessment, interpretation and planning, and intervention. Each of these three chapters ends with a 200-question practice test that exclusively reviews the material in that particular content outline. Appendix C contains a 200-question comprehensive examination; the answers to this exam are located in Appendix E.

For additional examination practice, as well as practice with the computer interface, this book contains a *200-question practice examination on computer disk*. Rationales are provided for these questions. These questions can be randomized several times, thus allowing repeated examination practice.

The references utilized for the test-item construction are those most commonly used in entry-level professional curricula; thus, they are contemporary and relevant for practice. To recent graduates of education programs in the United States, the references will be familiar. For those educated outside of the United States and those who are returning to the profession after 5 or more years' absence, this book will provide a comprehensive view of contemporary practice. Lists of these references are provided at the end of each chapter; additional sources for review are listed in Appendix D.

The questions in this book focus on problem-solving and thus are comparable to those on the actual licensure examination. However, these exams should not be reviewed as replicates of actual licensing examinations, nor should the reader attempt to memorize them.

How to Use this Book

Prospective test-takers will find this text useful for identifying areas of strengths and areas in which additional study is required. By reviewing the overall picture of entry-level physical therapy practice in Chapter 1, you will become familiar with the breadth and depth of practice requirements. Then, by reviewing each of the three major components of practice (i.e., assessment, interpretation and planning, and intervention), you should be able to quickly identify areas of your knowledge that do or do not require additional focused study. You can quickly note these findings on special "self-assessment" pages located at the back of each chapter. After you read each chapter, you can take the practice tests to confirm which content areas require additional study.

Once you have identified areas for additional review, check the reference list at the end of the chapters to identify those books and articles that are relevant to your further study. After you have read these references, you should go back and repeat the examinations at the end of the chapters. If there are still some areas of weakness, re-review the references to find the correct responses to the test items you missed.

After you have successfully completed the three chapter examinations, take the comprehensive examination in Appendix C and compare your answers with those in Appendix E. For each question you missed, ask yourself, "Why is that the best answer? Why are my choice and the other possible answers not correct?" If the answer does not readily emerge, go back to the references to validate why the correct answer is the only or most encompassing, accurate response.

When you are comfortable with the written tests, proceed to the computerized examination. Once you have completed the examination, the computer program will allow you to compare your choices with the actual answers. Rationales are provided. In addition, the program will show you which content area each question covers, thus pointing you toward any areas where you need more review. Once you have reviewed your references again, retake the computer examination to check your improvement—the computer will automatically shuffle the questions for you.

This computerized examination not only provides another opportunity for you to practice answering questions, but it will also familiarize you with how computerized examinations work. There is a big difference between looking down at a page of questions and looking forward at a computer screen that displays one question at a time. Successfully completing computerized examinations require certain skills, and learning these skills now will play a major part in reducing your anxiety on test day.

The contributing test writers and I hope that this book will assist you in passing the licensure examination. We further hope that this text will be evidence of the continuing evolution of physical therapy practice in the United States.

Patricia Rae Evans

Acknowledgments

I wish to express my profound gratitude to my colleagues and students at Samuel Merritt College, who continually challenged me to write this book and who enabled me to complete it in the 20th century.

I am also continually humbled by the support of Jean-François Vilain and Christa Fratantoro of F. A. Davis Company, who gently and persistently encouraged and insisted from day one to the completion of this decadelong project. I will always remember them with gratitude and friendship.

Diane Allen, MS, PT
Adjunct Assistant Professor
Samuel Merritt College
Oakland, California

*Evaluation, Diagnosis, and Management
of Clients with Neurological Dysfunctions*

Linnette Clark, MS, PT
Assistant Professor
Samuel Merritt College
Oakland, California

*Evaluation, Diagnosis, and Management
of Clients with Musculoskeletal Dysfunctions*

Patricia Rae Evans, MEd, PT
Associate Professor
Samuel Merritt College
Oakland, California

*Bioethics; Legal Aspects of Practice;
Delivery Systems; Research Design and
Statistics; Theories of Learning and
Motivation*

Mary Edna Harrell, MS, PT
Adjunct Faculty
Samuel Merritt College
Oakland, California

*Evaluation, Diagnosis, and Management
of Clients with Musculoskeletal
Dysfunctions*

Martha J. Jewell, PhD, PT
Professor
Samuel Merritt College
Oakland, California

*Anatomy; Biomechanics; Kinesiology;
Neuroanatomy; Pathology; General
Medicine*

Terrence Nordstrom, MS, PT
Assistant Professor
Samuel Merritt College
Oakland, California

Administration and Management

David Selkowitz, MS, PT
Assistant Professor
Samuel Merritt College
Oakland, California

*Evaluation, Diagnosis, and Management
of Clients with Musculoskeletal and
Neurological Dysfunctions*

Don Sokolski, MS, PT
Adjunct Faculty
Samuel Merritt College
Oakland, California

*Evaluation, Diagnosis, and Management
of Clients with Cardiopulmonary
Dysfunctions*

Linda Treml, MHS, PT
Adjunct Faculty
Samuel Merritt College
Oakland, California

*Case Management; Managed Care;
Oncology; Proprioceptive Neuromuscular
Facilitation Techniques*

Gail Widener, PhD, PT
Associate Professor
Samuel Merritt College
Oakland, California

*Physiology; Exercise; Physiology; Pathology;
Neurophysiology; General Medicine*

Lynn A. Colby, MS, PT
Assistant Professor Emeritus
Ohio State University
Physical Therapy Division
Columbus, Ohio

Mark W. Cornwall, PhD, PT, CPed
Associate Professor
Department of Physical Therapy
Northern Arizona University
Flagstaff, Arizona

Joan Edelstein, MA, PT
Director, Program in Physical Therapy
Associate Professor of Clinical Physical
    Therapy
Columbia University
New York, New York

Ginge Kettenbach, MS, PT
Assistant Professor
Department of Physical Therapy
Saint Louis University
St. Louis, Missouri

Edmund M. Kosmahl, EdD, PT
Associate Professor
Department of Physical Therapy
University of Scranton
Scranton, Pennsylvania

Joseph McCulloch, PhD, PT
Professor and Head
Department of Physical Therapy and
    Rehabilitation
Louisiana State University Medical Center
Shreveport, Louisiana

Roger M. Nelson, PT, PhD, FAPTA
Professor and Chair
Department of Physical Therapy
Thomas Jefferson University
Philadelphia, Pennsylvania

Cynthia C. Norkin, EdD, PT
Professor Emerita
College of Health and Human Services
School of Physical Therapy
Ohio University
Athens, Ohio

Jan F. Perry, EdD, PT
Professor and Chair
Department of Physical Therapy
School of Allied Health
Medical College of Georgia
Augusta, Georgia

Thomas J. Schmitz, PhD, PT
Associate Professor
Division of Physical Therapy
Long Island University—Brooklyn Campus
Brooklyn, New York

R. Scott Ward, PhD, PT
Associate Professor and Co-Director
Division of Physical Therapy
University of Utah
Salt Lake City, Utah

Elizabeth L. Weiss, PhD, PT
Professor and Director
Department of Physical Therapy
Louisiana State University Medical Center
New Orleans, Louisiana

Mary Ann Wilmarth, MS, PT, OCS
Assistant Clinical Specialist Faculty
Department of Physical Therapy
Northeastern University
Andover, Massachusetts

Contents

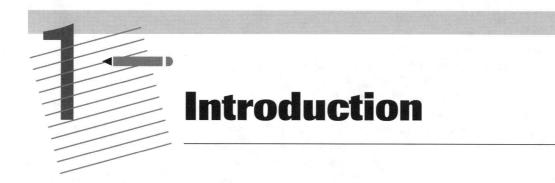

Introduction

This chapter includes an overview of state licensure policies, the licensure examination, and the purpose and use of the book. It also provides an introduction to problem-based multiple choice test items, computer-based examinations, general study guides, and strategies for preparing for the physical therapist licensure examination in the United States, the District of Columbia, and Puerto Rico. States, territories, and the District of Columbia are referred to as "the legal jurisdictions" throughout the rest of the book.

LICENSURE

The legal requirements for practicing physical therapy are established by the individual legal jurisdiction. Eligibility criteria for licensure, although similar, vary from jurisdiction to jurisdiction. Generally the initial criterion is the educational preparation of the individual. Typically, individuals must provide evidence of graduation from a professional program accredited by the Commission on Accreditation in Physical Therapy Education (CAPTE) or its predecessors. CAPTE has authority to accredit education programs. The requirements for internationally educated individuals who have graduated from non–CAPTE-accredited programs are unique to the legal jurisdiction in which an individual wishes to obtain licensure. The requirement of successful completion of the written physical therapist licensure examination is constant in all legal jurisdictions. This national examination is administered by the individual states, the District of Columbia, and Puerto Rico. There may be additional requirements imposed by the states. For example, a supplemental examination addressing the Physical Therapy Practice Act is required in California. A typical requirement for graduates from professional programs outside the United States is evaluation of the individual's academic preparation to determine educational equivalency. This is done by a recognized credentials evaluation service. Each legal jurisdiction provides applicants with the names of several approved evaluation services. Not all states accept evaluations from the same agencies. Foreign-educated therapists may also be required to successfully complete a specified period of supervised clinical experience in an approved clinical setting. Information regarding the specific licensure requirements for physical therapists and the application process in a legal jurisdiction can be obtained from the respective physical therapy board. A list of physical therapy boards is included in Appendix A.

OVERVIEW

Chapters 2 to 4 reflect the content areas of the current physical therapist licensure examination structure as established by the Federation of State Boards of Physical Therapy (FSBPT). The appendixes include a list of addresses of the licensing boards and the Federation, a glossary of terms, a comprehensive 200-item multiple choice examination, a selected bibliography, and answers to the comprehensive examination items.

Each of the examination content chapters begins with an outline of the clinical competencies and knowledge, skills, and attitudes inherent to clinical practice. The outlines were developed after an extensive analysis of practice by the FSBPT and were first published in 1997. They are reproduced as distributed without editorial changes. A rationale for including the content is provided together with suggested readings for additional study. Approximately 200 multiple choice items are included in each of the content areas. Three or more sample questions precede the multiple choice items. The sample questions are explained from the perspective of which response is correct and why the remaining responses are incorrect. At the end of each chapter the reader is asked to identify his or her strengths in major content areas, the areas in which improvement is needed, and to create a learning plan by which to establish competence and comfort in responding to questions in the content area.

The multiple choice items included in Chapters 2 to 4 and Appendix C were developed by physical therapists with known expertise in the content area. The items reflect the type of questions included in the licensure examination; they are not intended to represent actual items from the examination. The questions are designed to provide practice using a problem-based multiple choice format and an opportunity to structure further study by identification of strengths and weaknesses.

The list of mailing addresses, telephone numbers, and fax numbers for the physical therapy licensing boards is included in Appendix A as a reference for obtaining licensure information in one or more legal jurisdictions. Because application requirements differ, it is essential to obtain information directly from the jurisdiction or jurisdictions in which practice is desired. Licensure in one legal jurisdiction does not automatically qualify a physical therapist for licensure in another jurisdiction. This is particularly relevant for therapists graduating from programs outside the United States that are not accredited by the CAPTE. It is also important for graduates of CAPTE-accredited programs who have not practiced for a number of years or have allowed their license to lapse for more than 5 years.

A glossary of terms reflecting acceptable terminology is provided in Appendix B because certain terms are fairly unique to the United States. Appendix C is a comprehensive 200-item written examination that is designed to provide practice using a problem-based multiple choice format. It is also useful in identifying the length of time required to complete a 200-item examination. Selecting a bibliography that includes major references used in domestic physical therapist professional programs is discussed in Appendix D. Appendix E contains the answers to the Comprehensive Multiple Choice Examination. Answers are included to provide feedback on performance.

PURPOSE

The contextual framework of this book enables the reader to focus study in preparation for the examination, practice testing through experiential exercises, and foster confidence in approaching computer-based examinations. In addition, the book provides a framework for assessing the individual's areas of strength and those in need of additional intense studying before registration for the licensure examination.

EXAMINATION STRUCTURE

In 1997, the FSBPT completed a comprehensive analysis of the practice of physical therapists. Data were collected from more than 8000 practicing clinicians. Based on this analysis new licensure examination content outlines for the national physical therapist examination were developed and disseminated.

The current physical therapist licensure examination consists of three interwoven major content areas: Assessment and Evaluation (24% of the examination), Interpretation and Planning (22%), and Intervention (54%). Copies of the test content outline and partial and full analyses from the comprehensive data collection for the physical therapist may be obtained for a nominal fee directly from the Federation of State Boards of Physical Therapy, 509 Wythe Street, Alexandria, VA 22314; phone: (703) 299-3100.

The actual licensure examination contains 200 multiple choice questions. The intent is to determine by written examination the competence of an individual as a physical therapist practitioner. In the United States, clinical specialization is at the postprofessional level and certification examinations are provided in a number of areas. The licensure examination is restricted to the knowledge, skills, and attitudes expected of physical therapist generalists who have graduated from professional programs.

The examination is primarily problem based instead of requiring rote memorization of facts and details. It requires higher cognitive functioning and integration of content at the synthesis, analysis, and evaluative levels. Consequently, foundational knowledge is required in the basic, clinical, behavioral, and social sciences; communication skills; management principles; ethical issues; legal principles; as well as in physical therapy evaluations, diagnostics, and interventions. Problem-based examinations require practitioners to reflect on and solve realistic patient problems. Clinical decision making is an integrative process that requires sound knowledge of foundational content, skillful interpretation of patient data, and the ability to logically and accurately analyze situations. It also requires strict adherence to ethical and legal principles historically based on the Hippocratic Oath, the Nuremberg Code, the Doctrine of Helsinki, the American Physical Therapy Association Code of Ethics, federal and state laws governing practice, civil laws regarding malpractice, and civil rights legislation. Although the purpose of state licensure is the protection of the citizens of the respective jurisdiction, true safety can only be assured if practitioners are aware of contemporary research, continually seek current competence, and understand and accept the responsibilities of being professionals. Therefore, the examination includes test items dealing with these areas.

According to the FSBPT, the distribution of the test items is currently 24% in Assessment and Evaluation, 22% in Interpretation and Planning, and 54% in Intervention. The distribution of test items in the subcontent areas is presented in the following table:

Section	Subcontent Area		Percentage of Examination Items
1. Assessment & Evaluation			24%
	General Procedures		
	Data Collection	7%	
	Tests & Measurements	11%	
	System Specific Procedures	6%	
2. Interpretation & Planning			22%
	Data Interpretation	13%	
	Goal Setting and Care Planning	9%	
3. Intervention			54%
	Preparation	10%	
	Implementation	23%	
	Education/Communication/ Consultation	7%	
	Supporting Activities	8%	
	System Specific Procedures	6%	

MULTIPLE CHOICE EXAMINATIONS

The multiple choice format for testing consists of an incomplete stem (i.e., question or statement) that is accurately completed with one of the choices provided. Typically there are four choices available for each root. Three of the choices are plausible, but only one is correct or more encompassing than the other possible responses.

The test taker is required to make critical decisions when considering each item. Identifying the correct response requires careful reading of each option to progressively eliminate the incorrect choices. For example, if the stem includes a partial statement, the test taker should finish the sentence and then look at the possible answers to find the one that is consistent with his or her response.

COMPUTER-BASED EXAMINATIONS

Computer-based examinations require both a cognitive and psychomotor adaptation for most test takers. Since their inception, pencil-and-paper tests were the norm for most educational programs and licensure examinations. Beginning in 1999, only computerized examinations will be given. The physical therapist licensure examination requires completion within a specific time period. Items may be tagged as not answered, allowing the test taker to return to any unanswered items before completing the examination. Answers may also be changed before completion. There are 220 testing centers nationwide and in Canada. The examination can be scheduled on days that are personally convenient. Appointments must be made in advance with the testing center.

Experience in using computers is strongly recommended before scheduling the examination. Test takers need to be familiar with the standard keyboard of a personal computer or Macintosh and competent in basic keyboard skills, particularly in using the keys that control scrolling, paging up and down, and deleting or replacing a highlighted answer. A considerable amount of time and energy will be wasted if the test taker is inexperienced in the use of computers. For an individual who has taken the majority of examinations in the traditional format of pencil and paper or even Scantron forms that can be read by a computer, adjusting to viewing a computer monitor and using a keyboard for responses requires practice. When an individual has had no experience with computers, it is strongly recommended that a computer skills class be taken. For visually impaired individuals, other arrangements will be made by the respective legal jurisdiction. Examinations can be given verbally and time limits can be extended.

WAITING FOR YOUR SCORE

Scoring of the examination is not immediate, and the length of time for acquiring results varies among the legal jurisdictions; notification may take as long as 8 weeks. A limited number of states may grant a temporary license to practice pending successful completion of the examination. Other states use a license applicant status for a period of time immediately preceding the examination and until the score is available. Individuals may not practice as physical therapists until the legal jurisdiction has recognized the practitioner by granting applicant status, a temporary license, or the actual license itself.

STUDY STRATEGIES FOR PREPARING FOR AND TAKING THE EXAMINATION

Effective study strategies vary according to the needs and learning styles of each individual. There are general strategies in the education literature that may be beneficial. Studying for the physical therapist licensure examination requires both depth of understanding of content and the ability to articulate clearly and comprehensively. Physical therapists must think logically and rationally and consider multiple points of view in order to solve clinically based problems.

For well-educated individuals, multiple choice examinations are often troublesome because the test taker considers more and more possibilities and reads far more into a question than was ever intended by the writer (e.g., "If this, then this—but if this, then that.") Avoiding this pitfall is essential while preparing for and actually taking the licensure examination.

Before reading the content chapters and completing the comprehensive examination, the test taker should identify in writing his or her perceived areas of strength and weakness. The test taker should review the content areas covered by the licensure examination, ask a series of questions about each content and subcontent area, and compare them to his or her list of perceived strengths and weaknesses. Which are congruent and which are not?

Visualize a client arriving in the practice setting for the first time. Ask yourself:

- What is required in a thorough initial screening?
- What data should be gathered, and how are they interpreted?
- What are the implications of the findings?
- What is the physical or movement dysfunction diagnosis?
- What are realistic goals for the client?
- Which interventions are appropriate?
- What should be included in the initial management of the dysfunction?
- Are there ethical principles and issues to be attended to, such as confidentiality, informed consent, justice, and truth-telling?
- What portion of the treatment interventions are appropriate and legal for delegation to an assistant or an aide?
- What are the requirements and provisions for physical therapy services under Medicare and Medicaid?
- Is the client's physical therapy subject to capitation or limited numbers of visits?

- What are the major physiological effects of aerobic exercise?
- What motor control and learning theories are prevalent in the literature today?
- Which upper extremity proprioceptive

neuromuscular facilitation pattern helps the client to feed him- or herself?
- When is a home exercise program appropriate and how is learning fostered?

Based on these questions, identify the areas in which additional study is needed. Also think about how and when learning is most comfortable:

- Is it easier to study alone or in a group?
- Are small group discussions helpful?
- Does hands-on work with others facilitate learning?
- Does observing a master clinician enhance learning?

All people have preferred learning styles; one style may be very comfortable for an individual and another less comfortable. Determine which style is most effective and use it to prepare for the licensure examination. There are several standardized tests, such as the Myers Briggs Trait Inventory (MBTI) and the Kolb Learning Styles Inventory, that can provide valuable information on learning style preferences.

DEVELOPING A PREPARATION STRATEGY

Develop a realistic time frame to systematically prepare for the examination. Integrate study with the clinical decision making required of:

- Evaluation and diagnosis of neuromusculoskeletal dysfunctions
- Determination of expected outcomes and plans of care
- Implementation of various interventions
- Delegation to, and supervision of, physical therapy assistants
- Adherence to ethical and legal princi-

ples established and expected by the profession, community, and governmental agencies
- Consideration of the cost-effectiveness of intervention
- Awareness of the psychosocial aspects of illness, injury, and disability

In selecting resources for study, review the reference list included in each chapter and the selected bibliography in Appendix D. These references were selected on the basis of their citations in the professional literature and their use in academic programs in the United States and the District of Columbia. If educated outside the United States and Canada or if returning to practice after a prolonged absence, review journal articles that have been published within the past 5 to 7 years.

Organize the resources to support study in the areas perceived to be deficient. This can be accomplished by developing an outline of the content areas that require concentrated study. List several questions that, when answered, will be evidence of competence. Next list five to ten references that will facilitate answering these questions. Do not become overly intent with trying to read all of the literature in any or all content areas; this is neither efficient nor possible.

Establish study days and times and keep them sacred. Establish starting and ending dates for studying in each of the content areas. Determine the sequence of the questions to be answered and establish the study strategy in concert with answering the questions sequentially.

During the month immediately preceding the examination, focus on the decision-making processes used when evaluating, diagnosing, planning, and implementing a plan of care. Again, identify areas of personal strengths and weaknesses within the decision-making process and systematically eliminate the areas of weakness. Review progress each week. As each of the questions on the list of weaknesses is answered, cross it off the list. As the list narrows, revise the plan to address each of the remaining items.

Review a single segment of content in one setting. Then engage in an internal mental dialogue with the major authors and master clinicians, asking, "What would the expert do if confronted with this situation?" Then answer from the perspective of the author or master. Don't overload in a study setting because it can reduce confidence and impede learning.

Personal learning style suggests a need to engage in dialogue. Ask other license applicants or peers to discuss the content and pose relevant questions. This helps to refine knowledge of content. Complete the comprehensive written examination in this book again to see if there is a difference in performance since the first time it was completed.

The evening before the examination should be relaxed and devoid of study. Get a reasonable amount of sleep and arrange to arrive early at the examination location. Most of all, believe in yourself. During the examination, pace yourself and anticipate the correct response to a test item. If you find that you have used the same letter (A, B, C, D) three or more times in a row, double check the questions to verify each answer. Generally, no letter is used more than twice in succession. Answer all of the questions because there is no penalty for guessing; only correct responses are recorded and used to determine the raw score and percentage score on the examination. Generally, it is a good practice not to change answers unless absolutely certain the marked response is wrong.

It is suggested that you consider the examination as a means by which to verify a knowledge base sufficient to allow safe and effective practice of physical therapy. The suggestions contained here are not exhaustive. Academic experience may have already identified effective and efficient study strategies; use the strategy that is most effective and efficient for you.

References

Evaluative Criteria for Accreditation of Physical Therapist Education Programs. Alexandria, VA, Commission on Accreditation of Physical Therapy Education, 1997.

LSI Learning-Style Inventory. Boston, McBer & Company, 1993.

PT and PTA Analysis of Practice Reports, Alexandria, VA, Federation of State Boards of Physical Therapy, March 12, 1997.

Notes

Assessment and Evaluation

In 1997 the Federation of State Boards of Physical Therapy identified the following test content under the rubric of Assessment and Evaluation. Please note that throughout the content outlines, competence statements are the basis of the multiple choice questions. Note also that a number of subsets recur throughout the test content outline; this is an indication of the importance of the item or activity as it transects multiple activities. Twenty-four percent of the test items are devoted to demonstrating competence in assessment and evaluation; this means that approximately 48 items directly address the ability to collect data, show knowledge of both general and specific tests, and use measurements commonly used by physical therapists in the United States.

GENERAL PROCEDURES

Data Collection

Obtain the following patient information and interpret implications for education:

Medical/surgical history
- Interpretation of relevant information from the medical record
- How to seek information related to the chief complaint, behavior of source of the complaint, aggravating and relieving factors, history of the complaint, medical history, social history during interview
- Determination if client's signs/symptoms are indicative of local and/or systemic origin
- Evaluation of published studies related to PT practice

Special tests and diagnostic procedures (e.g., angiography, stress test, arthrogram, pulmonary functions tests, roentgenogram, CT, MRI reports sonograms, and electrocardiography)
- Interpretation of relevant information from the medical record
- How to seek information related to the chief complaint, behavior of source of the complaint, aggravating and relieving factors, history of the complaint, medical history, social history during interview

- Determination if client's signs/symptoms are indicative of local and/or systemic origin
- Evaluation of published studies related to PT practice

Medications
- Interpretation of relevant information from the medical record
- How to seek information related to the chief complaint, behavior of source of the complaint, aggravating and relieving factors, history of the complaint, medical history, social history during interview
- Major classes of drugs used in the treatment of musculoskeletal, neurological, cardiovascular, respiratory, and dermal systems
- Determination if client's signs/symptoms are indicative of local and/or systemic origin
- Evaluation of published studies related to PT practice

Laboratory results
- Interpretation of relevant information from the medical record
- How to seek information related to the

chief complaint, behavior of source of the complaint, aggravating and relieving factors, history of the complaint, medical history, social history during interview
- Determination whether client's signs/symptoms are indicative of local and/or systemic origin
- Mechanisms, rationale, and techniques to reduce the potential for transmission of infection

Psychosocial history and current status
- Interpretation of relevant information from the medical record
- How to seek information related to the chief complaint, behavior of source of

the complaint, aggravating and relieving factors, history of the complaint, medical history, social history during interview

Home environment, family and community support systems
- Interpretation of relevant information from the medical record
- How to seek information related to the chief complaint, behavior of source of the complaint, aggravating and relieving factors, history of the complaint, medical history, social history during interview
- Resources that may assist clients and families

Test/Measurements

Perform selected physical therapy assessments in a safe and accurate manner including handling all monitoring devices, equipment, or lines attached to or around patient
- How to inform clients regarding the purpose and methods of a procedure, what to expect, and what is expected from them
- Purpose of each assessment
- Selection of appropriate evaluation tools
- Positioning of the client to ensure safety, comfort, modesty, and effectiveness of intervention
- Purposes and precautions of client monitoring and support equipment including mechanical ventilators, pulse oximeter, suction, IV lines, ECG, urinary catheters
- Adapting body positions, movements, and equipment to prevent and/or reduce injuries to self
- Evaluation of published studies related to PT practice

Select and justify evaluation procedures and applications that are appropriate to the patient's status, medical diagnosis, treatment, age, functional needs, and any limiting factors
- Purpose of each assessment procedure
- Human anatomy and physiology
- Interpretation of relevant information from the medical record
- How to seek information related to the chief complaint, behavior of source of the complaint, aggravating and relieving factors, history of the complaint, medical history, social history during interview

- Selection of appropriate evaluation tools
- Provocation tests
- Determination if client's signs/symptoms are indicative of local and/or systemic origin
- Health-care delivery system

Observe the patient's response to the physical therapy assessment and treatment procedures and respond accordingly
- Recognition of signs of physiological distress
- Psychosocial stressors that may affect client response to pain
- Concepts of human growth and development from conception to senescence, including physical, cognitive, social, and emotional development
- Normal and abnormal psychology
- Clinical signs and symptoms of common psychiatric disorders
- How to alter activities in response to client response
- Major classes of drugs used in the treatment of musculoskeletal, neurological, cardiovascular, respiratory, and dermal systems
- Recognition of allergic reactions to treatment
- Determination if client's signs/symptoms are indicative of local and/or systemic origin

Determine patient need for assistive devices (e.g., positional supports or mobility aids)
- Positional changes or changes in ambulation and wheelchair mobility
- Wound status and signs of inflammation and/or healing

- Identification of normal and abnormal posture
- Static/dynamic balance tests in sitting/standing/movement patterns
- Abnormal reflex patterns
- How to integrate findings of multiple tests to clarify the client's problem and functional status
- How to determine the assistance the client requires during functional activities
- Use of devices such as bolsters, balls, and cylinders
- Resources that may assist clients and families

Perform reevaluations based on changes in patient status as appropriate
- Scientific and theoretical basis for various treatments
- Effects of various treatments
- How to alter activities in response to client response
- Recognition of allergic reactions to treatment
- Determination if client's signs/symptoms are indicative of local and/or systemic origin

Evaluate balance and coordination
- How to provide challenges to static/dynamic balance
- Interaction between visual, vestibular, and proprioceptive systems
- Static/dynamic balance tests in sitting/standing/movement patterns
- Appropriate vestibular techniques
- Differentiation of dysfunction between components of balance

Evaluate pain
- Administration and interpretation of pain scales
- Psychosocial stressors that may affect client response to pain

Evaluate functional mobility
- Positional changes or changes in ambulation and wheelchair mobility
- Purpose, structure, content, and demonstration of use of various functional tests
- How to observe clients' performances of graded functional tasks

Evaluate endurance
- Monitoring of heart, breath, and voice sounds
- Recognition of signs of physiological distress
- Application of target heart rate knowledge to client activities
- Substitution patterns and synergy patterns

- How to observe clients' performances of graded functional tasks

Determine client need for therapeutic seating or wheelchairs
- Positional changes or changes in ambulation and wheelchair mobility
- Wound status and signs of inflammation and/or healing
- Identification of normal and abnormal posture
- Use of devices such as bolsters, balls, and cylinders

Evaluate functional capacity
- Positional changes or changes in ambulation and wheelchair mobility
- Performance of flexibility tests
- Factors that affect muscle performance
- Psychosocial stressors that may affect client response to pain
- Substitution patterns and synergy patterns
- How to observe client's performance of graded functional tasks
- How to integrate findings of multiple tests to clarify the client's problem and functional status

Evaluate cognitive function as it relates to client's participation in PT program and attainment of goals
- How to question client appropriately to assess cognitive status relative to safety, judgment, and reasoning
- Concepts of human growth and development from conception to senescence, including physical, cognitive, social, and emotional development
- Normal and abnormal psychology
- Clinical signs and symptoms of common psychiatric disorders

Perform sensory/perceptual testing
- Appropriate techniques for tactile, proprioceptive, and vestibular sensory testing
- Techniques to perform a cranial nerve examination
- Differentiation between peripheral, dermatomal, and central sensory deficit

Perform structure-specific tests (e.g., vertebral impingement syndromes)
- Human anatomy and physiology
- Provocation tests
- Appropriate handling techniques to obtain accurate client response
- Differentiation between peripheral, dermatomal, and central sensory deficit
- Differentiation between peripheral, myotomal, and central motor deficits

Evaluate gait
- Positional changes or changes in ambulation and wheelchair mobility
- Determination of whether postural or gait deviations are appropriate adaptations or potentially harmful
- Identification of normal and abnormal gait
- Underlying impairments that contribute to gait deviations

Perform manual muscle testing
- Human anatomy and physiology
- Factors that affect muscle performance
- Appropriate handling techniques to obtain accurate client response
- Techniques and parameters of manual muscle testing
- Determination and control of substitution
- Correct performance of myotomal vs. prime mover tests
- Muscle actions, prime movers, and innervations

Evaluate muscle performance (e.g., with equipment, isokinetics, substitution, etc.)
- Factors that effect muscle performance
- Correct application of instrument to measure muscle force

- Determination and control of substitutions
- How to read instruments appropriately to measure muscle force
- Muscle actions, prime movers, and innervations

Identify normal and abnormal postures
- Human anatomy and physiology
- Identification of normal and abnormal posture

Measure joint range of motion
- Human anatomy and physiology
- Appropriateness of a device and the correct alignment to measure joint range of motion
- Osteo- and arthrokinematics for all joints
- Correct active and passive movement of body parts through range of motion at various speeds to assess tone or joint range of motion
- Capsular patterns of joint restrictions

Measure length and girth of body parts
- Landmarks used for length and girth measurements
- Correct application of tape measure along or around body parts to measure girth or length

SYSTEM-SPECIFIC PROCEDURES

Measure blood pressure and pulse rate during rest and exercise
- How to inform clients regarding the purpose and methods of a procedure, what to expect, and what is expected from them
- Human anatomy and physiology
- Selection of appropriate evaluation tools
- Proper stethoscope use
- Correct application of sphygmomanometer cuff to client's arm, inflation of cuff and ability to listen to Korotkoff sounds
- Location and palpation of arterial pulses with fingertips

Evaluate circulatory status
- Purpose of each assessment procedure
- Human anatomy and physiology
- Selection of appropriate evaluation tools
- Tests of peripheral circulation
- Location and palpation of arterial pulses with fingertips
- Recognition of signs of physiological distress

- Recognition of deviations from normal heart rhythms and breathing patterns

Evaluate status of musculoskeletal structures, soft tissue, integrity, muscle tone, joint play and flexibility
- Purpose of each assessment procedure
- Human anatomy and physiology
- Techniques to palpate soft tissue to determine tone, and soft tissue integrity
- Grades of and tests for accessory joint motion
- Provocation tests
- Tests of joint integrity
- Osteo- and arthrokinematics for all joints
- Correct active and passive movement of body parts through range of motion at various speeds to assess tone or joint range of motion
- Capsular patterns of joint restrictions
- Determination if client's signs/symptoms are indicative of local and/or systemic origin

Evaluate status of skin (e.g., wounds/burns)
- Human anatomy and physiology

- Skin color and integrity and pattern of hair growth
- Techniques to palpate skin to assess temperature, moisture, turgor, and texture
- Wound status and signs of inflammation and/or healing
- Determination if client's signs/symptoms are indicative of local and/or systemic origin
- Mechanisms, rationale, and techniques to reduce the potential for transmission of infection

Evaluate pulmonary status (e.g., chest mobility, auscultation, percussion, cough, sputum)

- How to inform clients regarding the purpose and methods of a procedure, what to expect, and what is expected from them
- Human anatomy and physiology
- Selection of appropriate evaluation tools
- Proper stethoscope use
- Monitoring of heart, breath, and voice sounds
- Recognition of signs of physiological distress
- Correct positioning of hands for chest percussion to evaluate lung density
- Purposes and precautions of client monitoring and support equipment including mechanical ventilators, pulse oximeter, suction, IV lines, ECG, urinary catheters
- How to attach and remove an oxygen saturation monitor
- How to palpate thorax for normal and abnormal signs
- How to place hands on chest to assess chest motion
- Recognition of deviations from normal heart rhythms and breathing patterns
- Determination whether client's signs/symptoms are indicative of local and/or systemic origin
- Mechanisms, rationale, and techniques to reduce the potential for transmission of infection

Identify heart sounds and changes

- Human anatomy and physiology
- Selection of appropriate evaluation tools
- Proper stethoscope use
- Monitoring of hearts, breath, and voice sounds
- Recognition of deviations from normal heart rhythms and breathing patterns

- Determination if client's signs/symptoms are indicative of local and/or systemic origin

Identify client need for orthotic or prosthetic devices

- Landmarks used for length and girth measurement
- Correct application of tape measure along or around body parts to measure girth or length
- Purpose of each assessment procedure
- Human anatomy and physiology
- Factors that affect muscle performance
- Prescription, fabrication, and use of adaptive devices
- Resources that may assist clients and families

Evaluate movement patterns and motor output control

- Substitution patterns and synergy patterns
- Abnormal reflex patterns
- Identification of appropriate sites for electrode placement
- How to position client to elicit primitive reflexes such as Babinski, cremaster, abdominal reflexes

Perform electrodiagnostic test

- Correct insertion of needles in client's muscle for electrodiagnostic testing
- Electrophysiology
- Characteristics of electrical stimuli
- Correct selection and preparation of electrodes and skin for application of electrodes to client's skin
- Identification of appropriate sites for electrode placement
- Determination if client's signs/symptoms are indicative of local and/or systemic origin

Evaluate neurologic status (central and peripheral and autonomic)

- Human anatomy and physiology
- Anatomy and physiology of reflex mechanisms
- Location of appropriate sites for electrode placement
- Determination if client's signs/symptoms are indicative of local and/or systemic origin

Evaluate achievement of developmental milestones in pediatric clients

- Appropriate age onset/integration of reflexes and milestones
- Test for developmental milestones

- Concepts of human growth and development from conception to senescence, including physical, cognitive, social, and emotional development

- How to position client to elicit primitive reflexes such as Babinski, cremaster, abdominal reflexes

INTENT OF CONTENT SECTION

One of the major roles of physical therapists is to evaluate and diagnose movement dysfunctions and musculoskeletal and neurologic disorders. On the examination, these items represent an integration of anatomy, physiology, neuroanatomy, neurophysiology, lifespan considerations, clinical decision making, and screening processes; evaluation procedures; diagnosis of movement dysfunctions and musculoskeletal disorders. Knowledge of the underlying material; clinical, applied, behavioral, and social sciences; and the professional procedures and approaches used by physical therapists are inherent to screening, evaluation, and diagnosis processes.

Items that reflect this content area require knowledge, comprehension, application, synthesis, analysis, and evaluation of information. Examples of test items in this content area include:

EXAMPLE #1:

A 15-year-old boy is referred for evaluation of an inability to resume playing tennis 8 weeks after fracture of the radial head. The initial evaluation should obtain objective data regarding:

A. level of tennis playing in which patient is engaged
B. activities that cannot be performed
C. range of motion and muscle strength
D. expectations of the client and family

The correct response is C. The stem of the item requested identification of *objective* data that should be obtained; A, B, and D reflect subjective reporting. Although this information may likely be obtained, it is not objective in nature.

EXAMPLE #2:

When walking up an incline, the pelvis tends to assume a position of _____, which requires correction to maintain a neutral position in the lumbar area.

A. anterior tilt
B. lateral tilt
C. rotation
D. posterior tilt

The correct response is D. This item requires using of biomechanical principles to ascertain changes in forces and torque experienced while ascending an incline. Visualizing the activity is an important test-taking strategy and should occur before selecting a response.

EXAMPLE #3:

An elderly client gets around the house with a front-wheeled walker. His daughter takes him grocery shopping because he needs help descending stairs at the front of the house. A front-wheeled walker is used at the grocery store with the daughter standing by. During shopping at the mall, a wheelchair is used. The client is:

A. an unlimited community ambulator
B. an independent limited community ambulator
C. an assisted limited community ambulator
D. an independent household ambulator

The correct response is C. By carefully reading the narrative, it is clear that this client always has assistance when ambulating. It is also clear that ambulation does occur part of the time. Therefore, the key words are "assisted" and "limited." Careful reading of examination items often is the determining factor in selecting the correct response.

SAMPLE TEST ITEMS COVERING ASSESSMENT AND EVALUATION CONTENT

Please read the stem of each item carefully. Without looking at the possible choices, formulate the answer to the question or complete the statement. Then carefully look for the correct response in the choices provided. If a response cannot be selected, place a mark by the item and return to it after all of the sample questions have been answered. Then go back to the marked items and try again. If the answer still remains illusive, star the item and write the number in the notes page. Develop a study question that will facilitate answering the question. The correct answers are included at the end of the chapter.

1. **A physiological or accessory movement:**

   A. can exceed the anatomical limit of a motion
   B. can be performed within the pathological limit of motion
   C. cannot be performed beyond the pathological limit
   D. can be performed in all fibrous joints

2. **A client fell off a horse and complains of left knee pain and numbness and tingling on the lateral aspects of both thighs. What type of neurologic examination is indicated?**

   A. CNS because the common peroneal nerve may be damaged
   B. PNS because the common peroneal nerve may be damaged
   C. CNS because present history and symptoms indicated possible spinal cord compression
   D. PNS because the symptoms are inferior to the gluteal fold

3. **A 14-year-old boy comes to your clinic complaining of pain on the bottom of the heel of the left lower extremity that he got when playing basketball. The client plays basketball 6 days a week for at least 1 or 2 hours a day and plays on two league teams. On examination the client describes pain when the lateral edges of his heel are squeezed. The nature of the problem is most likely:**

   A. Achilles tendinitis
   B. Sever's disease
   C. Achilles bursitis
   D. calcaneal stress fracture

4. **A construction worker complains of pain in the left knee after standing all day. To relieve this pain, the leg must be elevated for 1 hour. What information indicates severity?**

   A. elevation for 1 hour required to relieve pain
   B. the existence of pain in the left knee
   C. the client's occupation
   D. work requires prolonged standing

5. **In performing a musculoskeletal evaluation, a result of "strong and painful" refers to a:**

   A. neurologic strength test
   B. static or isometric strength test
   C. manual muscle test
   D. functional muscle test

6. **A result of "Fair+" means that the muscle tested was able to complete:**

   A. the full range of motion against gravity with no resistance
   B. the entire range of motion against gravity with a little resistance
   C. some but not all the range of motion against gravity, no resistance
   D. all the range of motion with gravity eliminated with a little resistance

7. **According to several research articles regarding the clinical reliability of manual muscle testing (MMT):**

   A. MMT has poor inter-tester reliability on grades below Fair
   B. staff physical therapists can perform MMT reliably in a clinical setting
   C. physical therapists are reliable with half a grade
   D. using dynamometers is not any more reliable than MMT

8. **Positive results on which one of the following tests is consistent with posterolateral knee instability?**

   A. posterior drawer and anterior drawer
   B. posterior drawer and varus stress
   C. posterior drawer and valgus stress
   D. extension and abduction accessory test

9. **The most effective approach to differentially diagnosing among plantar fascitis, Achilles bursitis, and Achilles tenonitis is:**

   A. palpation
   B. active dorsiflexion with toe extension
   C. the box test, especially dorsiflexion inversion
   D. passive physiological movement of dorsiflexion, G IV++

10. **The correct way to document hip joint measurement of 90 degrees of flexion and lacking 10 degrees of extension from neutral is:**

    A. -10–90
    B. Flex: 0–90; Ext: 0–10
    C. 10-0–90
    D. 10–90

11. **Which one of the following statements is true about a capsular pattern of range-of-motion limitation?**

    A. It does not involve a fixed number of degrees for each motion but rather a fixed proportion of one motion relative to another motion.
    B. It is usually caused by a condition involving structures such as ligament shortening, muscle strains, and muscle contractures.
    C. It usually involves only one or two motions of a joint in contrast to noncapsular patterns that involve all or most motions of a joint.
    D. Joints in which their movements have more firm end-feels tend to develop capsular patterns.

12. **All of the following are examples of closed kinetic chain activities except:**

    A. pushup
    B. bench press
    C. stairclimb
    D. lunge

13. **Which of the following is not a mechanism by which nosocomial infections can be transmitted?**

    A. inadequate hand washing
    B. equipment not cleaned between patient use
    C. exposure to an individual with chicken pox
    D. contamination from bandage scissors

14. **Which one of the following is a normal blood pressure response to exercise?**

    A. Systolic pressure remains the same during active exercise.
    B. Systolic pressure returns to the normal resting value 15 to 20 minutes after exercising.
    C. Systolic pressure gradually increases with exercise, plateaus as the exercise intensity plateaus, and declines as exercise intensity declines.
    D. Diastolic pressure increases more than 10 to 15 mm Hg during the exercise or activity.

15. **When taking blood pressure, the first sound heard is:**

    A. ventricular relaxation
    B. the diastolic pressure
    C. Korotkoff's sound phase III
    D. the systolic pressure

16. **A 29-year-old woman who delivered her third child 1 month ago complains of pain from the right PSIS to the right PIIS and sometimes midline in the groin region. The back pain started when she was about 7 or 8 months pregnant and is aggravated by walking (heel strike with right lower extremity) and going down stairs and curbs leading with her right leg. The pubic pain started soon after delivery and is aggravated by the same activities as the sacral pain, but occurs only when the sacral pain is a 6 on a 10-point analog scale. The disorder consistent with these findings is:**

    A. a groin pull secondary to the delivery position
    B. hypermobility (instability) of the pelvic joints secondary to a hormone released during pregnancy
    C. hypermobility of the pelvic joints secondary to the stresses placed on them during delivery
    D. postpartum stress disorder

17. **This type of contraction occurs when the force of the muscle is less than the resistance:**

    A. concentric
    B. eccentric
    C. isometric
    D. isokinetic

18. **The part of the primary motor cortex that controls movement of the thigh is supplied by the:**

    A. anterior cerebral
    B. middle cerebral
    C. posterior cerebral
    D. anterior and middle cerebral
    E. middle and posterior cerebral

19. **A posterior central herniation of the L2–3 disc could irritate and/or compress the:**

    A. dorsal columns of the spinal cord
    B. anterior spinal artery
    C. conus medullaris
    D. L2 root unilaterally
    E. S2–4 roots bilaterally

20. **A patient has a medical diagnosis of poliomyelitis. Which of the following do you expect to find on evaluation?**

    A. hyperactive deep tendon reflexes
    B. spotty sensory deficits
    C. spotty muscle weakness
    D. spasticity
    E. all of the above

21. **If a patient is unable to dorsiflex past the neutral position, there would be a problem with all of the following except:**

    A. shock absorption at the ankle
    B. ascending stairs
    C. forward progression
    D. stability

22. **Stride length is:**

    A. the linear distance between the right and left steps
    B. normally 14 to 20 inches or 35 to 50 cm
    C. decreased in the elderly population
    D. also measured by doubling the step length

23. **A shoulder quadrant test should be performed:**

    A. every time passive mobility testing for the shoulder is performed
    B. if the patient has no pain on other passive mobility tests
    C. to assess laxity for a patient with chronic shoulder pain
    D. if the patient has pain on passive glenohumeral flexion or abduction

24. **If a patient has restricted shoulder abduction that is equal for both active range of motion and passive range of motion, the restriction would most likely be due to:**

    A. deltoid muscle weakness
    B. supraspinatus tendinitis
    C. superior capsule tightness
    D. latissimus dorsi tightness.

25. **A 20-year-old collegiate swimmer presents with left anterior shoulder pain. During freestyle swimming, pain increases when the shoulder is in maximum flexion and extension and internal rotation are initiated. The patient is unable to maintain sidelying on the shoulder and is unable to abduct through an arc of 90 to 120 degrees without pain. The highest pain level occurs with a combination of end-range flexion with internal rotation. The mostly likely diagnosis is:**

    A. posterior shoulder instability
    B. acromioclavicular joint arthritis
    C. rotator cuff strain
    D. an impingement syndrome

26. **All of the following can refer pain to the shoulder except the:**

    A. elbow
    B. spleen
    C. liver
    D. lung

27. **In assessing range of motion in cervical lateral flexion to the left:**

    A. the normal range of motion is 65 degrees
    B. align the fulcrum of the goniometer with the occipital protuberance
    C. measure from the middle of the chin to the left acromion process with a tape measure
    D. stabilize the right shoulder girdle to prevent lateral flexion of the thoracic and lumbar spine

28. **A client complains of dizziness when looking over his right shoulder while backing his car out of the driveway. A vertebral artery test:**

    A. should be done if performing a G.II to the cervical spine
    B. would be positive if the client had a symptom of facial paresthesia
    C. would be performed if the client had passive range of motion of cervical rotation to 30 degrees on the right.
    D. would only be indicated if the client also complained of dizziness with other activities involving cervical rotation

29. **Upper cervical stability testing is:**

    A. always performed before any mid- to lower cervical mobilization
    B. imperative to perform when a patient has a history of ankylosing spondylitis
    C. necessary to perform when all cervical movements are severely limited
    D. only necessary to perform when a computed tomography scan shows an odontoid fracture

30. **The typical presentation of carpal tunnel syndrome may include all of the following except:**

    A. awakening at night due to fourth and fifth digit pain or tingling
    B. atrophy of the thenar eminence
    C. wrist and hand pain
    D. higher incidence with pregnancy

31. **All of the following are true about sensation testing except:**

    A. two-point discrimination is not helpful in identifying early-stage nerve compression
    B. 2 to 5 mm is considered normal for adults in two-point discrimination in the hand
    C. the Semmes-Winstein test is an example of a threshold test
    D. threshold tests are not useful in detecting nerve compression or postsurgical recovery

32. **In order to evaluate edema in the hand, the therapist can use:**

    A. a volumeter
    B. circumferential measurements
    C. visual inspection
    D. all of the above

33. **Which of the following procedures is most commonly used to determine activity tolerance after myocardial infarction?**

    A. graded exercise test (GXT)
    B. percutaneous transluminal coronary angioplasty (PTCA)
    C. echocardiography
    D. cardiac angiogram

34. **A client with insulin-dependent diabetes mellitus is referred for evaluation. In the chart review it would be consistent with the medical diagnosis to find abnormally high amounts of:**

    A. lipids
    B. cholesterol
    C. glucose
    D. all of the above
    E. B and C only

35. **All of the following are true about computed tomography (CT) scanning except:**

    A. CT scans use x-rays to project an image.
    B. CT scans can directly image axial cross sections of the body.
    C. CT scans can directly image sagittal sections of the body.
    D. CT scans are effective for assessing bone density.

36. **The advantage of performing a myelogram over a plain radiograph is a myelogram:**

    A. allows direct visualization of the spinal cord and radiographs do not
    B. allows visualization of the "thecal" (dural) sac and radiographs do not
    C. allows visualization of all surrounding soft tissues and radiographs do not
    D. shows areas of increased cellular activity indicating areas of inflammation and radiographs do not

37. **A female client reports a 10-week history of morning stiffness lasting 2 to 3 hours, symmetric joint swelling in her ankles and knees, and bilateral hand pain. These symptoms are probably early signs of:**

    A. scleroderma
    B. systemic lupus erythematosus
    C. osteoarthritis
    D. rheumatoid arthritis
    E. gout

38. **Which type of scaphoid fracture is prone to delayed healing?**

    A. distal pole fracture
    B. waist fracture
    C. proximal pole fracture
    D. tuberosity fracture
    E. neck fracture

39. **A 27-year-old client complains of night pain in both wrists and paresthesias along the volar aspect of the thumb and index, middle, and half of her ring fingers. Which splint is most appropriate for relief of pain and numbness?**

    A. a pneumatic cuff
    B. a long-arm splint with the elbow flexed less than 90 degrees
    C. a hand-based thumb spica splint
    D. a wrist extension splint with the wrist in 20 to 30 degrees extension
    E. a wrist splint with the wrist in the neutral position

40. **All of the following are true about benign tumors except:**

    A. They are slow growing.
    B. They are well defined and have a demarcated sclerotic ring.
    C. They do not metastasize.
    D. They are generally highly invasive of the surrounding tissues.

41. **A 45-year-old client complains of fatigue and diffuse musculoskeletal pain associated with multiple areas of tenderness throughout her body. The clinical features are consistent with:**

    A. fibromyalgia
    B. thoracic outlet syndrome
    C. lupus
    D. Reiter's syndrome

42. **A client presents with a diagnosis of thoracic outlet syndrome (TOS). To rule out cervical nerve root involvement, which of the following tests should be performed?**

    A. Roos test
    B. slump test
    C. Adson's test
    D. foraminal compression test
    E. upper limb tension test

43. **If collagen breakdown is allowed to exceed the collagen formation as in a repetitive strain injury, the condition will become chronic. This pathological process is consistent with that of all of the following except:**

    A. medial epicondylitis
    B. rotator cuff tendinitis
    C. tenosynovitis
    D. lateral epicondylitis
    E. all of the above follow this pathology

44. **A 27-year-old client reports enlarged axillary and cervical lymph nodes for the past month. The client presents with a fever and complains of fatigue and weight loss. Questioning and physical examination reveal no evidence of joint pain or visible skin changes. The most appropriate action at this point is to:**

    A. continue with a more extensive objective evaluation
    B. refer the client to a primary care physician
    C. begin a treatment program of active range-of-motion and active assistance range-of-motion exercises
    D. include cryotherapy as a part of your treatment approach

45. **A 25-year-old client complains of a recent episode of low back pain. Radiograms show narrowing of the SI joint spaces and squaring of the anterior borders of the thoracic and lumbar vertebrae. The diagnosis is:**

    A. nerve root impingement
    B. ankylosing spondylitis
    C. spondylolisthesis
    D. degenerative disk disease

46. **Thoracic outlet syndrome (TOS) can result from all of the following except:**

    A. a cervical rib
    B. a scalene minimus muscle
    C. a large callous from a healed clavicular fracture
    D. prolonged overhead work
    E. all of the above can lead to TOS

47. **Reflex sympathetic dystrophy is characterized by all of the following except:**

    A. pain and edema
    B. sympathetic nodules
    C. vasomotor abnormalities
    D. trophic changes
    E. all of the above

48. **A client has a tumor affecting the intermediate lobe of the spinocerebellum. What dysfunction may be present during the initial evaluation?**

    A. difficulty initiating limb movements
    B. difficulty with the execution of movement
    C. difficulty learning new motor tasks
    D. uncoordinated limb movements while in the supine position

49. **One of the tests you use in your assessment of a neonate is rooting reflex assessment. You administer this test by:**

    A. stroking the upper lip and waiting for the lip to retract
    B. using a finger to lightly stroke the corner of the infant's mouth
    C. using a finger to firmly apply pressure to the corner of the infant's mouth
    D. any of the above

50. **During your assessment of an 8-month-old neonate, you observe the asymmetrical tonic neck reflex (ATNR). This may be indicative of:**

    A. athetosis
    B. central nervous system damage
    C. normal development
    D. any of the above

51. **A child with central nervous system damage becomes agitated when positioned prone. This may be caused by:**

    A. the lack of spontaneous extension drive with consequent difficulty in lifting the head in order to clear the airway
    B. increased ATNR with resulting rotation to one side
    C. the root reflex interfering with breathing
    D. the moro reflex being triggered more frequently

52. **A 23-year-old client suffered a spinal cord injury while rock climbing and is independent in transfers with assistive devices. The spinal cord level involved is below:**

    A. C5
    B. C6
    C. C7
    D. T1

53. **A client has been referred for evaluation of a possible peripheral nerve injury. A nerve conduction velocity (NCV) test is performed. The rationale is that the NCV can:**

    A. be used for treatment purposes as well as diagnosis
    B. pinpoint the location of the suspected nerve entrapment
    C. provide prognostic as well as diagnostic data
    D. isolate the cause of injury

54. **A 35-year-old client is referred by a rheumatologist for evaluation and treatment. Consultations with a variety of physicians yielded no diagnosis until examination by the rheumatologist. The medical diagnosis is fibromyalgia. The client probably:**

    A. is very satisfied with the health-care system
    B. will focus the dialogue on anything but the symptoms
    C. has issues similar to persons with disabilities after primary neurologic disorders
    D. will appreciate validation when the condition is termed psychosomatic

55. **The main problems for a 70-year-old client with Parkinson's disease can be expected to include all of the following except:**

    A. decreased balance
    B. bradykinesia
    C. kyphotic posture
    D. hypotonicity

56. **When performing a subjective evaluation of an 82-year-old client in acute inpatient care after a right cerebrovascular accident, it is important to:**

    A. get information from the chart only because the patient may be unreliable
    B. allow the patient time to respond because cognitive processing may be slowed
    C. defer obtaining information pertaining to the home environment
    D. address only items that can be factually substantiated

57. **When assessing movement control using the Fugl-Meyer assessment, all of the following are necessary except:**

    A. providing clear verbal instructions, miming the movement if necessary
    B. asking the patient to repeat the movement three times and score on best performance
    C. facilitating the movement if the patient has difficulty
    D. having the client perform the movement with the unaffected limb first

58. **A 30-year-old client is referred for evaluation of low back pain. Symptoms cannot be reproduced during the objective evaluation. The client requests four bathroom breaks during the 45-minute evaluation and complains of increased low back pain upon returning each time. This behavior is consistent with:**

    A. stenosis
    B. cystitis
    C. nerve root irritation
    D. stress disorders

59. **An 80-year-old client is edematous, has flaky skin and a protruding abdomen, and is very apathetic. A cause of these symptoms may be:**

    A. vitamin C deficiency
    B. vitamin D overabundance
    C. kwashiorkor
    D. Ca^{++} deficiency

60. **A client presents with signs and symptoms associated with anemia caused by iron deficiency. These signs and symptoms are also like those seen in individuals with:**

    A. dementia
    B. multiple sclerosis
    C. myocardial ischemia
    D. cerebrovascular accident

61. **A very high hemoglobin level may indicate:**

    A. polycythemia
    B. sickle cell disease
    C. hemophilia B
    D. Hodgkin's disease

62. **A 69-year-old woman complains of back pain after performing extension movements during the evaluation. Which of the following subjective complaints is most indicative of an osteoporotic fracture?**

    A. pain radiating into the buttock and leg unilaterally
    B. constant pain not relieved by changing positions
    C. forward flexion of the trunk reduces her pain
    D. there was no history of trauma before the onset

63. **Distinguishing fibromyalgia from a mechanical dysfunction is based on:**

    A. extremity pain that radiates from distal to proximal
    B. trigger-point pain with radiation to a distal area
    C. dermatomal pain distribution
    D. all of the above

64. **Ankylosing spondylitis may be difficult to diagnose because:**

    A. it has an insidious onset
    B. the symptoms may be mild and non-progressive
    C. the symptoms can be confused with mechanical low back dysfunction
    D. all of the above
    E. B and C

65. **A client is referred for evaluation and management of chronic obstructive pulmonary disease (COPD) sequelae. The chart includes findings that are not consistent with COPD. Which of the following values are within normal limits?**

    A. $FVC = 3.1$ L; $FEV_1 = 1.4$ L
    B. $FVC = 2.9$ L; $FEV_1 = 2.7$ L
    C. $FVC = 5.1$ L; $FEV_1 = 4.1$ L
    D. $FVC = 2.6$ L; $FEV_1 = 5.2$ L

66. **Pitting edema of both feet may be a sign of:**

    A. cor pulmonale
    B. pneumonia
    C. atelectasis
    D. excess activity

67. **Breath sounds are normally heard at the:**

    A. left lateral ribcage
    B. sternum
    C. manubrium
    D. heart

68. **An advantage of a tracheotomy in a ventilator-dependent patient is that it:**

    A. increases the dead air space
    B. increases the residual volume
    C. allows the patient to eat
    D. all of the above

69. The chest radiographs for a client who sustained a cerebrovascular accident reveal blunting of the right costophrenic angle. This is most likely due to:

    A. pneumothorax
    B. pleural effusion
    C. right upper lobe pneumonia
    D. left lower lobe atelectasis

70. The most common source of a pulmonary embolus is:

    A. pleural effusion
    B. pulmonary edema
    C. hemothorax
    D. deep vein thrombosis

71. In the third session with a client recovering from a mild cerebrovascular accident, the client is supine. Respiratory rate is 40 RPM. Left ankle and leg edema with a positive Homan's sign. Temperature is 98.6°F. The most likely cause of the observed tachypnea is:

    A. cor pulmonale
    B. pulmonary embolus
    C. pneumonia
    D. emphysema

72. When assessing a client's respiratory rate, it:

    A. may be measured by placing the hand on the client's diaphragm and ribcage
    B. may be measured for 10 seconds
    C. should be taken only after explaining the procedure to the patient
    D. may be measured by placing the hand on the lateral aspect of the last two ribs

73. The following information has been obtained during a discharge evaluation of a client with chronic obstructive pulmonary disease: (1) the client lives alone and a neighbor helps with meals; (2) he ambulated short distances independently before admission; (3) saturation of arterial blood with oxygen (SaO_2) at rest on 2 L oxygen by nasal cannula is 97%; (4) he ambulated independently slowly on room air for 50 ft; (5) is mildly short of breath and fatigued after walking; (6) SaO_2 on room air after ambulation is 92%. Which of the following would be the most appropriate discharge plan?

    A. home with supplemental oxygen and instructions on energy conservation techniques
    B. home without supplemental oxygen and with instructions on energy conservation techniques
    C. skilled nursing facility for physical therapy with supplemental oxygen and instructions on energy conservation techniques
    D. confine to bed with instructions on energy conservation techniques

74. Subjective and objective evaluations require documentation of your findings. Critical to the documentation of the objective evaluation is/are:

    A. active range-of-motion measurements
    B. cause of the injury
    C. client's psychological status
    D. statement of functional limitations

75. Which of the following would indicate a need to incorporate a nerve conduction velocity (NCV) test as part of an objective evaluation?

    A. progressive numbness and weakness ulnar nerve distribution
    B. increasing radiating pain posteromedial aspect proximal forearm
    C. postsurgical repair rupture long head of biceps brachii
    D. decreasing ability to perform overhead tasks

76. The study of motion is referred to as:

A. kinetics
B. kinematics
C. dynamics
D. statics

77. Percent change in shape is referred to as:

A. strain
B. viscoelasticity
C. stress
D. porosity

78. Passive joint distraction or traction is an example of what kind of force system?

A. linear
B. bending
C. concurrent
D. parallel

79. Passive joint distraction produces what kind of motion?

A. rotary
B. curvilinear
C. shear
D. translatory

80. The tibialis anterior functions as a _____ class lever during a concentric contraction in an open kinematic chain.

A. first
B. second
C. third
D. fourth

81. A client is prone and attempting trunk raises as a part of the functional assessment. The instruction is to hold the back in neutral as part of an evaluation of the strength of the gluteus maximus. During the concentric part of this activity, the gluteus maximus is functioning as a _____ class lever as it extends the hip.

A. first
B. second
C. third
D. fourth

82. A wall squat is requested as part of an assessment of a client's functional capacity. In the going-down phase of the squat, the vastus medialis functions as a _____ class lever.

A. first
B. second
C. third
D. fourth

83. In which lever system does the effort force always have the greatest mechanical advantage?

A. first
B. second
C. third
D. fourth

84. Which of the following does not occur in aging bone?

A. decreased brittleness
B. decreased stiffness
C. decreased total volume
D. decreased cross-sectional area

85. Which of the following structures has the greatest maximum possible porosity?

A. tendon
B. cortical bone
C. cancellous bone
D. articular cartilage

86. In articular cartilage, the _____ zone has the greatest porosity.

A. superficial tangential
B. middle
C. deep
D. subcontral

87. There is continued deformation with a constant or maintained load. This best describes which of the following?

A. Wolff's law
B. injury
C. stress-relaxation
D. creep

88. **Strength decreases in normal aging of collagenous dense regular connective tissue. This is caused by or contributed to by all of the following except:**

    A. decreased fiber diameter
    B. decreased number of nonreducible cross bridges
    C. decreased stiffness
    D. decreased total collagen

89. **Which of the following provides both mechanical strength and a diffusion barrier to the axons it surrounds?**

    A. epimysium
    B. perimysium
    C. endomysium
    D. none of the above

90. **Axon function can be compromised by compression or tension and sometimes both. Compression and tension affect axon function by:**

    A. causing the axon to depolarize prematurely
    B. causing mechanical distortion of the myelin sheath
    C. decreasing circulation
    D. separating the terminal button from the motor endplate at the synaptic junction

91. **Which type of muscles are better at producing range of motion than they in producing force?**

    A. multipennate
    B. unipennate
    C. strap
    D. bipennate

92. **Which type of contraction occurs when the origins and insertions of the contracting muscle are brought closer together because of the action of the muscle?**

    A. concentric
    B. eccentric
    C. isometric
    D. isokinetic

93. **A client may be asked to perform a muscle-setting exercise as part of the objective evaluation. This type of exercise consists of:**

    A. contracting a skeletal muscle for 5 seconds without moving the associated body part
    B. alternately contracting and relaxing a skeletal muscle without moving the associated body part
    C. contracting a skeletal muscle and moving the associated body part through the range of motion
    D. alternately contracting and relaxing a skeletal muscle and moving the associated body part

94. **Recruitment order has to do with the order in which:**

    A. muscle cells are recruited in an individual motor unit
    B. individual collagen fibers in a tendon are recruited
    C. motor units are recruited during muscle contraction
    D. individual collagen fibers in a ligament are recruited

95. **What kind of lubrication is described as a monolayer absorbed to the surface of the articular cartilage and is dependent on chemical, not physical, properties of the molecule?**

    A. hydrodynamic
    B. hydrostatic
    C. squeeze film
    D. boundary

96. **The ability of tissue to regain its original shape and size after being stretched or otherwise deformed is referred to as:**

    A. plasticity
    B. elasticity
    C. viscoelasticity
    D. contractility

97. In a concentric contraction, velocity is _____ related to load.

A. directly
B. inversely
C. never
D. maximally

98. Degeneration of articular cartilage is related to all of the following except:

A. changes in the collagen (increased number of fixed cross links)
B. excessive stress concentration
C. magnitude of the stresses
D. number of stress peaks

99. The hypoglossal nerve exits through the _____.

A. spinal cord
B. medulla
C. pons
D. midbrain

100. In which structure(s) is/are the vestibular nucleus located?

A. medulla
B. pons
C. midbrain
D. medulla and pons

101. Ganglion is to the peripheral nervous system as _____ is to the central nervous system.

A. neurophil
B. neuron
C. capsule
D. cortex

102. Which of the following are unmyelinated axons?

A. C fibers
B. A delta fibers
C. preganglionic autonomic motor fibers
D. B fibers

103. The part of the primary motor cortex that controls movement of the thigh is supplied by which of the following arteries?

A. anterior cerebral
B. middle cerebral
C. posterior cerebral
D. anterior and middle cerebral

104. Which of the following will have the fastest conduction velocity?

A. group II fiber
B. afferent from the Golgi tendon organ
C. A-gamma fiber
D. preganglionic autonomic motor fiber

105. A thrombus in a branch of the _____ artery may affect the pyramids.

A. anterior spinal
B. basilar
C. vertebral
D. posterior spinal

106. Typically when someone refers to the central nervous system and uses the term "hemisphere," the reference is to the:

A. lateral half of the cerebrum or the cerebellum
B. medial half of the frontal lobe
C. lateral half of the temporal lobe
D. medial half of the parietal lobe

107. Afferents from the facial, glossopharyngeal, and vagal nerves are received by the:

A. nucleus ambiguus
B. nucleus solitarius
C. salivatory nucleus
D. vestibular nucleus

108. In the brainstem, _____ links cranial nerve nuclei that control extraocular muscles with the vestibular nucleus

    A. medial vestibulospinal tract
    B. lateral lemniscus
    C. medial lemniscus
    D. lateral vestibulospinal tract

109. A lesion in the left area could result in an inability to recognize:

    A. voices
    B. tactile stimuli
    C. written words
    D. melodies

110. A client has a medical diagnosis of syringomyelia. Which of the following can be expected on evaluation?

    A. bilateral hyperactive deep tendon reflexes in the lower extremities
    B. contralateral loss of fine motor control
    C. A and C
    D. A and B

111. The cranial nerve(s) that supply the muscles of the tongue is/are:

    A. III, IV, and VI
    B. XII
    C. V
    D. VII

112. Which of the following is a sign of cerebellar disease?

    A. tremor at rest
    B. akinesia
    C. athetosis
    D. ataxia
    E. alexia

113. Sensory innervation for olfaction is provided by which cranial nerve?

    A. I
    B. III
    C. V
    D. VII

114. Indications for stopping an exercise test include all of the following except:

    A. the systolic blood pressure reaches 210 mm Hg
    B. the subject requests that the test be stopped
    C. an increase or decrease in the S-T segment of the electrocardiogram pattern
    D. multifocal premature ventricular contractions

115. During electrodiagnostic testing of a client with a suspected peripheral nerve injury, the number of action potentials generated can be best increased by:

    A. decreasing the ramp time
    B. increasing the rise time
    C. increasing the ramp time
    D. increasing the frequency

116. Electrical stimulation is often a part of the evaluation for clients presenting with weakness of the left extensor carpi radialis. Of the following choice, which one has been shown to stimulate the most forceful contractions?

    A. beat-modulated alternating current
    B. straight, unmodulated alternating current
    C. monophasic pulsatile current
    D. biphasic, symmetrical, pulsatile current

117. If during a neurologic evaluation there is a decrease in sensation in the C8 dermatome, which one of the following muscle groups would be manually tested?

    A. flexor carpi ulnaris, extensor carpi ulnaris, third and fourth lumbricals
    B. supinator, flexor digitorum profundus, first and second lumbricals
    C. extensor carpi radialis longus, extensor indices, first and second lumbricals
    D. brachioradialis, extensor digitorum, flexor carpi ulnaris, third and fourth lumbricals

118. **A 30-year-old client who is 5′ 10″ and weighs 220 lbs has a sudden onset of pain in the right lumbar area radiating into the buttock while lifting heavy objects and turning to the left. He was unable to return to a neutral position. These findings are consistent with a:**

    A. bulging low lumbar disc
    B. blocked low lumbar facet
    C. lumbar paraspinal muscle strain
    D. degenerative upper lumbar disc irritating nerve root

119. **For the client described in item 118, which of the following would be most appropriate and necessary to determine the exact nature of the movement dysfunction in the objective examination?**

    A. stop movements short of provoking low back and buttock pain
    B. determine the limit of active range of motion (AROM) or passive range of motion (PROM) that produces low back and buttock pain
    C. have client perform movements to the end of the available AROM or PROM and apply overpressure
    D. encourage movement to the point of provoking lower extremity pain

120. **For the client in item 118, which of the following objective tests is the least likely to reproduce pain?**

    A. forward bending in standing
    B. right-side bending in standing
    C. manual traction in the supine position
    D. repeated flexion in the supine position

121. **The purpose of the heel-knee test is to:**

    A. determine active range of motion
    B. assess functional ability
    C. rule out degenerative disc disease
    D. assess coordination of movement of extremities

122. **An individual with _____ shows the first signs of the condition when he is in his 40s.**

    A. Hutchinson's disease
    B. rheumatoid arthritis
    C. Huntington's chorea
    D. multiple sclerosis

123. **The cranial nerve that provides for sensory innervation to the middle ear is the:**

    A. trochlear
    B. glossopharyngeal
    C. vagus
    D. vestibulocochlear

124. **A brisk contraction of a muscle in response to a sudden stretch induced by a sharp tap on the tendon of insertion is the definition of a/an:**

    A. abnormal reflex
    B. spastic condition
    C. deep tendon reflex
    D. denervated muscle

125. **_____ is a recessive genetic metabolic disorder characterized by pellagra-like skin lesions, transient cerebellar ataxia, and hyperaminoaciduria.**

    A. Hashimoto's disease
    B. Hartnup disease
    C. Hansen's disease
    D. Hers' disease

126. **The induction phase is the:**

    A. period of time during which a normal cell becomes transformed into a cancerous cell
    B. analysis of data and examination of practice problems within their own contexts
    C. amount of time required for a muscle to respond to an electrical stimulus
    D. process of stimulating and determining morphogenetic differentiation in a developing embryo

127. **A disease characterized by muscle atrophy caused by degeneration of the anterior horn cells of the spinal cord and primarily affecting the upper extremities is:**

    A. amyotrophic lateral sclerosis
    B. Duchenne-Erb paralysis
    C. multiple sclerosis
    D. Duchenne-Aran disease

128. **The F wave recorded in electroneuromyographic testing appears on _____ stimulation of a motor nerve and is caused by antidromic transmission of a stimulus.**

    A. submaximal
    B. supramaximal
    C. subminimal
    D. minimal

129. **The element in the human body that helps regulate neuromuscular excitability and muscle contraction is:**

    A. carbon dioxide
    B. oxygen
    C. potassium
    D. copper

130. **An area on the surface of a body innervated by afferent fibers from one spinal root is a:**

    A. dermatome
    B. myotome
    C. sensory distribution pattern
    D. peripheral nerve pattern

131. **A normal neural reflex elicited by touching the soft palate or posterior pharynx is referred to as the:**

    A. swallowing reflex
    B. pursed-lip reflex
    C. gag reflex
    D. laryngeal reflex

132. **The condition involving inflammation of a tendon sheath caused by calcium deposits, repeated strain or trauma, or high levels of blood cholesterol is:**

    A. tendinitis
    B. tenosynovitis
    C. myositis
    D. chondromyelitis

133. **A Trendelenburg gait is an abnormal gait associated with a weakness of the _____ muscle.**

    A. iliopsoas
    B. gluteus maximus
    C. gluteus medius
    D. tensor fascia lata

134. **A client presents with a neurologic dysfunction. During the evaluation, fine, rhythmic, purposeless movements occur and increase during voluntary movements. These movements are:**

    A. continuous tremors
    B. intention tremors
    C. choreiform movements
    D. athetoid movements

135. **A client presents with a history of progressive inability to do bilateral toe raises. In the initial screening examination, which muscle should be tested?**

    A. anterior tibialis
    B. peroneus longus
    C. extensor hallucis longus
    D. gastrocnemius

136. **A client with a cardiac condition indicates the presence of stabbing or burning pain that is made worse by coughing, swallowing, deep breathing, and lying down. It is relieved by aspirin and other anti-inflammatory drugs. The pain described is referred to as:**

    A. pericardial pain
    B. pulmonary embolism pain
    C. myocardial ischemic pain
    D. pain arising from the great vessels

137. **In documenting the evaluation of a client with suspected pulmonary disease, the client's total volume of air within the chest after a maximum inspiration is recorded as the:**

    A. functional residual capacity (FRC)
    B. dynamic lung volume and flow rate (FEV)
    C. forced vital capacity (FVC)
    D. total lung capacity (TLC)

138. **Patients with restrictive pulmonary diseases typically demonstrate:**

    A. rapid and shallow breathing
    B. rapid and deep breathing
    C. slow and shallow breathing
    D. slow and deep breathing

139. **For a client with a suspected pulmonary dysfunction, the measurement recorded at the end of a normal expiration when all respiratory muscles are relaxed is the:**

    A. maximal inspiratory pressure (MIP)
    B. dynamic lung volume (DLV)
    C. functional residual capacity (FRC)
    D. forced vital capacity (FVC)

140. **In examining a client who reports joint pain "ballotting," the joint will:**

    A. determine the passive range of motion
    B. elicit the presence of fluid
    C. assess for increased heat over the joint
    D. determine the presence of crepitus

141. **Forceful lateral or medial bending is applied while extending the leg is a test for:**

    A. collateral ligament tears
    B. meniscus tears
    C. patellar dislocation or subluxation
    D. contractures

142. **Local signs of inflammation are important in differentiating inflammatory and noninflammatory processes. Among the typical local signs by which this distinction can be made are:**

    A. limitations in motion and decreased strength
    B. decreased sensation and strength
    C. restrictions in motion and pain
    D. increased heat and erythema

143. **_____ is primarily a disorder of hyaline cartilage and subchondral bone, although all tissues in and around involved joints are hypertrophic.**

    A. Psoriatic arthritis
    B. Osteoarthritis
    C. Infectious arthritis
    D. Osteomyelitis

144. **Which test is useful in determining if there is an Achilles tendon rupture?**

    A. anterior drawer test
    B. Thompson's test
    C. Kleiger test
    D. talar tilt test

145. **During initial screening of a client referred for pain management, the client reports increased pain, becomes emotional, and expresses hopelessness. The pain is described as constant, present 24 hours a day, and viselike over the vertex. The objective evaluation reveals no physical abnormalities. The etiology of the client's dysfunction may be:**

    A. muscle tension
    B. organic brain disease
    C. conversion hysteria
    D. vascular

146. A 49-year-old woman is referred for evaluation and management of hemiparesis that started 5 days earlier. Functional loss is moderate. History includes migraines associated with hormonal changes and start of menses. The paresis is consistent with a/an:

A. cerebrovascular accident
B. transient ischemic attack
C. aneurysm
D. hysteria conversion episode

147. A client who presents with a syndrome of sensory loss, muscle weakness and atrophy, decreased deep tendon reflexes, and vasomotor symptoms involving many nerves simultaneously will probably have a diagnosis of:

A. mononeuropathy
B. multiple mononeuropathy
C. polyneuropathy
D. multiple polyneuropathy

148. In evaluating a client with a skin disease, an erosion and an ulcer can be distinguished by describing the loss of:

A. the epidermis and at least part of the dermis
B. part or all of the epidermis
C. normal color and texture
D. sensation

149. A client is referred after excision of a lymphangioma. This is a/an:

A. malignant tumor involving the lymphatic system
B. soft, movable, subcutaneous nodule
C. elevated lesion composed of dilated, cystic lymphatic vessels
D. nodule composed of fibroblastic tissue

150. A client who is a soccer player reports pain in the anterior compartment muscles. Onset of symptoms began with pain at heel strike and has progressed to an inability to hold the forefoot up during foot descent and eccentric contractions. Findings are consistent with:

A. stress fractures
B. shin splints
C. tendinitis
D. myositis

151. Alterations in structures at any level of the neuroaxis that are destructive to neural tissue are referred to as:

A. anomalies
B. vascular accidents
C. tumors or abscesses
D. lesions

152. As cranial and spinal nerves exit the dural sac, they acquire sheaths of meningeal dura called the:

A. falx cerebri
B. epineurium
C. denticulate ligaments
D. tentorium cerebelli

153. The thin layer of connective tissue closely adherent to the surface of the brain and spinal cord is the:

A. pia
B. arachnoid
C. dura
D. meningeal structure

154. Injury of the _____ can lead to a radicular distribution of hypoesthesia or hyperesthesia and motor weakness

A. pons
B. medulla
C. spinal roots
D. infratentorial compartment

155. **A client presents with loss of proprioception and vibratory sensory loss from the body and face. This is consistent with a small abscess in the:**

    A. pons
    B. medulla
    C. spinal roots
    D. infratentorial compartment

156. **It is consistent with a small unilateral bleed in the _____ to observe ataxia, facial paralysis, and internal strabismus of the eye.**

    A. pons
    B. medulla
    C. spinal roots
    D. infratentorial compartment

157. **Deficits in the timing of muscle contractions such as loss of balance, swaying, staggering, and intention tremor are consistent with a tumor in the:**

    A. thalamus
    B. cerebellum
    C. cerebrum
    D. pons

158. **Alterations of cognitive functions, changes in awareness, and loss of memory are consistent with damage to the:**

    A. thalamus
    B. cerebellum
    C. cerebrum
    D. pons

159. **Large areas of damage to the _____ that affect the reticular activating system typically result in coma and death**

    A. thalamus
    B. cerebellum
    C. cerebrum
    D. pons

160. **Trauma to the _____ can result in hyperkinesia, intractable intense pain, memory loss, altered behavioral patterns, endocrine imbalances, and autonomic dysfunction.**

    A. thalamus
    B. cerebellum
    C. cerebrum
    D. pons

161. **The basilar artery is the union of the:**

    A. anterior cerebral artery and middle cerebral artery
    B. anterior and posterior spinal arteries and vertebral artery
    C. internal carotid arteries
    D. posterior cerebral arteries

162. **A client with a subdural hematoma can often be distinguished from one with intracranial bleeding by the:**

    A. immediate onset of symptoms after a traumatic insult to the cranium
    B. early and progressive sensory deficits
    C. lag time in the onset of neurologic signs
    D. progressive motor deficits

163. **The clinical deficit that results from an isolated lesion of the dorsal columns is:**

    A. astereognosis
    B. hemianopsia
    C. dysarthria
    D. aphasia

164. **An injury to the spinocerebellar fibers in the brainstem is associated with:**

    A. weakness and spasticity
    B. diminished sensation to pinprick, touch, and temperature
    C. flaccid paralysis of extremities
    D. dysmetria, ataxia, and a loss of position sense of the extremities

165. **A tumor affecting the spinothalamic tract or anterolateral tract will result in:**

    A. weakness and spasticity
    B. diminished sensation to pinprick, touch, and temperature
    C. flaccid paralysis of extremities
    D. dysmetria, ataxia, and a loss of position sense of the extremities

166. **The _____ tract is located between the spinal trigeminal complex and the anterolateral system. It contains fibers from the contralateral red nucleus traveling to the ventral horn of the cervical and thoracic spinal cord.**

    A. accessory nucleus
    B. ventral spinocerebellar
    C. rubrospinal
    D. medial longitudinal fasciculus

167. **Damage to the _____ results in denervation of the tongue. On evaluation, the client's tongue will deviate toward the side of the injury.**

    A. hypoglossal nucleus
    B. dorsal motor nucleus of the vagus
    C. internal arcuate fibers
    D. medial accessory inferior olive nucleus

168. **Trauma to the lateral aspect of the spinal cord or the inferior cerebellar peduncle may result in:**

    A. nystagmus, vertigo, and falling
    B. ataxia in the upper extremity on the side ipsilateral to the injury
    C. unsteady balance, nausea, and nystagmus
    D. loss of two-point discrimination, position, and vibratory sense

169. **A client presents with transient chorea, loss of pain and temperature sensation from the contralateral face and body, ipsilateral Horner's syndrome, and contralateral supranuclear facial palsy. These symptoms are consistent with:**

    A. a lesion of the anterior inferior cerebellar artery
    B. infarction of the superior cerebellar artery
    C. infarction of the posterior inferior cerebellar artery
    D. damage to the red nucleus

170. **Complete bilateral deafness after an automobile accident in which a client sustains a closed-head injury is consistent with an injury of the:**

    A. superior cerebellar peduncle
    B. inferior colliculus
    C. lateral lemniscus
    D. superior colliculus

171. **The symptoms associated with total paralysis of the oculomotor nerve are:**

    A. double vision
    B. blindness
    C. loss of peripheral vision
    D. ptosis in ipsilateral eye

172. **A client with a diagnosis of Parkinson's disease will experience hypokinesia and bradykinesia. This syndrome involves neurodegeneration of the:**

    A. lateral geniculate
    B. pulvinar nucleus
    C. cerebral peduncle
    D. dopamine-containing neurons in the substantia nigra

173. **Tumors of the pineal gland produce upgaze palsy. The syndrome is named:**

    A. Parinaud's syndrome
    B. Benedikt's syndrome
    C. Weber's syndrome
    D. top of the basilar syndrome

174. **Clients with a medical diagnosis of a lenticular fasciculus tumor may present with which symptoms?**

    A. loss of appetite, emaciation, adipsia, and apathy
    B. sudden, unexpected chorealike or dystonic movements of the contralateral limbs
    C. fever, shivers, and chills
    D. amnesia, aphasia, and choreiform movements

175. **A client demonstrates spasticity and hemiplegia on the contralateral side with involvement of the upper extremity only. These findings are consistent with involvement of the:**

    A. temporal lobe
    B. postcentral gyrus
    C. lateral portion of the precentral gyrus
    D. occipital lobe

176. **A 70-year-old client presents in the emergency room with a history of hypertension, sudden onset pain on the right side of the head behind the ear, left-sided weakness, blood pressure of 200/112 mm Hg, respiration of 16 RPM, pulse rate of 88 BPM, left homonymous hemianopsia, and is awake and oriented. These signs and symptoms are consistent with a vascular accident in the:**

    A. posterior cerebral artery
    B. internal carotid artery
    C. middle cerebral artery
    D. anterior spinal artery

177. **A 68-year-old, left-handed client was referred for evaluation of progressive weakness and atrophy of both lower extremities over the past 9 months. Upper extremities and speech are also involved. She is awake and oriented with full visual fields, normal facial expression, deep tendon reflexes elevated at her knees and ankles and depressed at elbows and wrists. She has significant atrophy of all extremities. Widespread fasciculations are noted at rest in all extremities. She is able to rise from a chair and ambulate a short distance independently. Upper extremity tremor is present with shoulder flexion to 90 degrees and forearms pronated. Tremor is alleviated when upper extremities are in the neutral resting position. Her speech is slurred and her tongue protruded on the midline but weak; fasciculations are present on the surface of the tongue. Corneal, jaw-jerk, and gag reflexes are present but sluggish. Discriminative touch, vibratory sense, proprioception, and pain and temperature sensation are all intact, and her vital signs are within normal limits. Based on this information, at what level in the central neuraxis is the client's disorder?**

    A. upper brainstem
    B. lower brainstem and spinal cord
    C. frontal and parietal lobes
    D. left cerebral hemisphere

178. **For the client described in item 177, the pathology is:**

    A. not determinable
    B. focal
    C. multifocal
    D. diffuse

179. **For the client described in item 177, what is the clinical temporal profile of this pathology?**

    A. acute
    B. chronic
    C. progressive
    D. stable

180. **Why would a client demonstrate absence of pain and temperature sense on the left side and discriminatory touch and vibration on the right?**

    A. because of a mass-occupying lesion in the brainstem
    B. because of an injury to one side of the spinal cord
    C. because of a focal lesion in the medulla
    D. because of a bleed into the posterior cranial fossa

181. **A client has right-sided hemiparesis; homonymous hemianopsia; and disorientation with respect to time, place, and personal information. His speech is poorly articulated and perseverative. He has a 7-year history of hypertension. He has diabetes managed with insulin. His blood pressure is 180/100 mm Hg, and his heart rate and respiration are WNL. Muscle strength of the left extremities 5/5. RUE 3+/5. Right lower extremity, 4/5. Reflexes are normal on the left side. Deep tendon reflexes (DTR) elevated, RUE more so than right lower extremity. There is a positive Babinski sign. These findings are consistent with:**

    A. infarction involving either the thalamus or internal capsule
    B. trauma to left parietal lobe
    C. upper brainstem vascular hemorrhage
    D. space-occupying tumor in the midbrain

182. **The client described in item 181 should be:**

    A. referred back to the referring neurologist for additional workup
    B. evaluated to determine rehabilitation potential
    C. placed on a maintenance program until all medical conditions stabilize
    D. rescheduled for additional evaluative testing in 3 to 5 days

183. **A client presents with loss of tactile sensation; proprioception; vibration; two-point discrimination; graphesthesia; and stereognosis on the left side of the face, torso, and extremities. He has athetoid movements on his left hand with the eyes closed. He was diagnosed with myotonic dystrophy 5 years earlier. Initial evaluation reveals muscle weakness with marked atrophy of the proximal shoulder and hip musculature; and short-term memory loss. His condition is stable. Current signs and symptoms are consistent with:**

    A. the earlier diagnosis of myotonic dystrophy
    B. a vascular occlusion of the posterior choroidal and thalamolenticular arteries
    C. an infarction involving the right middle cerebral artery
    D. meningitis

184. **A 52-year-old client with right-sided hemiparesis, confusion, and aphasia was comatose for 2 days and progressively regained consciousness during the past week. Her sensation is intact, but she has a diminished right lower extremity. She has mild weakness in the right lower quadrant of her face and moderate weakness in her right extremities. She has elevated deep tendon reflexes, a positive Babinski sign, and bladder and bowel incontinence. She can read aloud but does not comprehend what she reads. She can follow single commands but not two- or three-step commands. She repeats single words when trying to answer questions. Her uvula is elevated on the midline and her tongue is protruded on the midline. Snout, grasp, and suck reflexes are absent. Her eyes tend to rest slightly to the left. These findings are consistent with:**

    A. anterior cerebral artery aneurysm
    B. supratentorial space-occupying lesion
    C. substance abuse or exposure to toxic agents
    D. trauma to the left temporal lobe

185. **A client referred for evaluation has a medical diagnosis of Parkinson's disease. Which of the following sets of symptoms is most consistent with this diagnosis?**

    A. decreased sensation, diplegic spasticity, and vertical nystagmus
    B. spasticity, retropulsion, and short-term memory loss
    C. intentional and resting tremors, bradykinesia, and postural embarrassment
    D. bradykinesia, resting tremor, retropulsion, and postural embarrassment

186. **Nine months ago a client developed rapid onset of right-sided hemiparesis and hemiparesthesia. Within 3 months, both symptoms resolved and ballistic movements developed in the right extremities. This is consistent with:**

    A. a second cerebrovascular hemorrhage
    B. progression of a slow bleeding aneurysm
    C. damage to the subthalamic nucleus
    D. involvement of the adjacent internal capsule

187. **The expected cognitive level of functioning of the client in item 186 is:**

    A. loss of orientation to person, time, and place
    B. not affected by the neurologic damage; therefore, intact and normal
    C. characterized by an inability to perform simple math processes
    D. not determinable secondary to probable aphasia

188. **The clinical profile of the pathology of the client in item 186 is:**

    A. acute
    B. chronic
    C. stable
    D. progressive

189. **A client is referred with a diagnosis of vascular hemorrhage with damage to the globus pallidus or pallidothalamic tracts. The clinical symptoms associated with this damage include:**

    A. left extremities involvement with preserved cognitive, memory, and language skills
    B. left extremities involvement with aphasia and memory loss
    C. right-sided athetosis and cognitive deficits
    D. right extremities involvement with preserved memory and language skills

190. **During the initial evaluation of a 38-year-old client referred for evaluation of movement dysfunctions resulting from a vascular accident, asynchronous vertical and horizontal nystagmus is observed as well as marked increased tone that is exacerbated by turning the head. The client is totally dependent in all activities of daily living. These findings are consistent with a lesion located in the:**

    A. posterior parietal area
    B. upper brainstem
    C. lower brainstem
    D. cerebral cortex

191. **A physical therapist is ethically required to refer a client to another physical therapist when:**

    A. the client requires evaluative or treatment services beyond the scope of the referring therapist
    B. the client requests a different therapist
    C. the therapist perceives a conflict of interest
    D. all of the above

192. **When evaluating a client with AIDS, health-care personnel must:**

    A. avoid exposure to bodily fluids
    B. frequently monitor the client's vital signs
    C. minimize any physical contact with the client
    D. address issues of pain management

193. **A client referred for evaluation of acute low back pain states that the pain is not relieved by lying down or by maintaining one position. This may indicate:**

    A. lumbar stenosis
    B. a visceral disease
    C. ankylosing spondylitis
    D. a space-occupying lesion

194. **A complaint of long-standing back pain that occurs at night and is not relieved by positional change indicates:**

    A. lumbar stenosis
    B. a visceral disease
    C. ankylosing spondylitis
    D. a space-occupying lesion

195. **Which of the following may ethically be delegated to a physical therapist assistant?**

    A. obtaining a client history
    B. sensory testing
    C. obtaining joint range-of-motion measurements
    D. performing a manual muscle test

196. **An appropriate task for a physical therapy aide to perform is:**

    A. obtaining an abbreviated client history
    B. setting up the treatment area
    C. obtaining joint range-of-motion measurements
    D. explaining the evaluation the physical therapist will perform

197. **If a client provides a copy of a physician's evaluation of a musculoskeletal condition, the physical therapist should:**

    A. conduct an evaluation and diagnose the movement dysfunction
    B. perform a screening examination
    C. forego an initial evaluation
    D. implement a treatment plan based on the physician's evaluation

198. **In the contemporary health-care environment, it is essential that after a client evaluation the physical therapist include in the documentation:**

    A. statements of functional outcomes
    B. only objective data
    C. pertinent information from the client's chart
    D. opinions regarding the client's probable medical diagnosis

199. **The condition that is a softening of bone secondary to impaired mineralization in the bone matrix is:**

    A. osteomyelitis
    B. osteomalacia
    C. osteoporosis
    D. osteosarcoma

200. **A client reported shoulder pain that is relieved by lying on the affected shoulder. This is a sign of:**

    A. subdeltoid bursitis
    B. thoracic outlet syndrome
    C. a radiculopathy
    D. a pulmonary cause of the pain

Correct Responses to Sample Items in Chapter 2

The following are the correct responses to items 1 to 200 contained in this chapter.

1. B	51. B	101. D	151. D
2. C	52. A	102. A	152. B
3. B	53. B	103. A	153. A
4. D	54. C	104. B	154. C
5. B	55. D	105. B	155. B
6. B	56. B	106. A	156. A
7. A	57. C	107. B	157. B
8. B	58. B	108. D	158. C
9. A	59. D	109. C	159. D
10. D	60. C	110. D	160. A
11. A	61. B	111. B	161. B
12. A	62. B	112. D	162. C
13. C	63. C	113. A	163. B
14. C	64. C	114. C	164. D
15. D	65. C	115. B	165. B
16. B	66. A	116. C	166. C
17. B	67. C	117. A	167. A
18. D	68. C	118. A	168. B
19. B	69. B	119. B	169. B
20. E	70. D	120. C	170. C
21. A	71. B	121. D	171. D
22. C	72. A	122. C	172. D
23. B	73. B	123. B	173. A
24. C	74. D	124. C	174. B
25. D	75. A	125. B	175. C
26. C	76. B	126. C	176. A
27. D	77. B	127. D	177. B
28. B	78. A	128. A	178. D
29. C	79. B	129. C	179. C
30. A	80. C	130. A	180. B
31. D	81. A	131. C	181. A
32. D	82. C	132. B	182. C
33. A	83. A	133. C	183. B
34. C	84. C	134. B	184. A
35. A	85. C	135. C	185. D
36. A	86. B	136. A	186. C
37. B	87. D	137. D	187. B
38. E	88. C	138. B	188. D
39. E	89. D	139. C	189. A
40. D	90. B	140. D	190. B
41. A	91. A	141. B	191. D
42. E	92. A	142. D	192. A
43. E	93. B	143. C	193. B
44. B	94. C	144. B	194. D
45. A	95. D	145. C	195. C
46. E	96. B	146. B	196. B
47. E	97. B	147. C	197. A
48. A	98. A	148. A	198. A
49. B	99. B	149. C	199. B
50. B	100. D	150. C	200. D

References

American College of Sports Medicine: Resource Manual for Guidelines for Exercise Testing and Prescription. Philadelphia, Lea & Febiger, 1988.

Barr, ML, and Kiernan, JA: The Human Nervous System. Philadelphia, JB Lippincott, 1993.

Bobath, B. Adult Hemiplegia: Evaluation and Treatment, ed 2. London, William Heinemann, 1979.

Boissonnault, WG: Examination in Physical Therapy Practice. New York, Churchill Livingstone, 1991.

Brannon, FJ, Foley, MW, Starr, JA, and Black, MG: Cardiopulmonary Rehabilitation: Basic Theory and Application. Philadelphia, FA Davis, 1993.

DeGroot, J, and Waxman, SG: Correlative Neuroanatomy, ed 22. Norwalk, CT, Lange Medical Publications, 1995.

Fiatarone, M, and Evans, W: The Etiology and Reversibility of Muscle Dysfunction in the Aged. J Gerontology 48:77–83.

Fugl-Meyer, AR, Jaasko, L, Leyman, I, et al.: The post-stroke hemiplegic patient: I. A method for evaluation of physical performance. Scand J Rehab Med 1975, 7:13–31.

Goodman, CC, and Snyder, TEK: Differential Diagnosis in Physical Therapy. Philadelphia, WB Saunders, 1995.

Hasson, SM: Clinical Exercise Physiology. St. Louis, Mosby, 1994.

Kandel, ER, Schwartz, JH, and Jessell, TM: Principles of Neural Science, ed 3. Elsevier, North Holland, 1991.

Kendall, F, McCreary, E, and Provanc, P: Muscles: Testing and Function, ed 4. Baltimore, Williams & Wilkins, 1993.

Lewis, C, Lindsay, T, and Scott, C: Functional Assessment in the Psychosocial Realm. Topics in Geriatric Rehab 11:64–83.

Magee, D: Orthopedic Physical Assessment, ed 2. Philadelphia, WB Saunders, 1992.

Maitland, GD: Peripheral Manipulation, ed 3. New York, Butterworth-Heinemann, 1991.

Maitland, GD: Vertebral Manipulation, ed 5. New York, Butterworth-Heinemann, 1986.

McArdle, WD, Katch, FI, and Katch, VL: Exercise Physiology: Energy, Nutrition and Human Performance, ed 3. Philadelphia, Lea & Febiger, 1993.

Moore, KL, and Persaud, TVN: Before We Are Born. Philadelphia, WB Saunders, 1993.

Moore, KL: Clinical Oriented Anatomy. Baltimore, Williams & Wilkins, 1992.

Netter, FM, and Colacino, S: Atlas of Human Anatomy. Summit, NJ, Ciba Medical, 1994.

Nordin, M, and Frankel, VH: Basic Biomechanics of the Musculoskeletal System. Philadelphia, Lea & Febiger, 1989.

Norkin, C, and Levangie, P: Joint Structure & Function. Philadelphia, FA Davis, 1992.

Norkin, C, and White, DL: Measurement of Joint Motion: A Guide to Goniometry, ed 2. Philadelphia, FA Davis, 1995.

O'Sullivan, SB, and Schmitz, TJ: Physical Rehabilitation: Assessment and Treatment, ed 3. Philadelphia, FA Davis, 1994.

Pierson, F: Principles and Techniques of Patient Care. Philadelphia, WB Saunders, 1994.

Robbins, SL, Cotran, RS, and Kumar, V: Pathological Basis of Disease, ed 2. Philadelphia, WB Saunders, 1995.

Rothstein, JM, and Echternach, JL: Primer on Measurement: An Introductory Guide to Measurement Issues. Alexandria, VA, American Physical Therapy Association, 1993.

Rothstein, JM, Roy, SH, and Wolf, SL: The Rehabilitation Specialist's Handbook. Philadelphia, FA Davis, 1991.

Sauerland, EK: Grant's Dissector. Baltimore, Williams & Wilkins, 1994.

Sawner, KA, and LaVigne, JM: Brunnstrom's Movement Therapy in Hemiplegia, ed 2. New York, JB Lippincott, 1992.

Schmidt, RA: Motor Learning and Performance. Champaign, IL, Human Kinetics Publishers, 1991.

Skinner, JS: Exercise Testing and Exercise Prescription for Special Cases: Theoretical Basis and Clinical Application, ed 2. Philadelphia, Lea & Febiger, 1993.

Umphred, DA: Neurological Rehabilitation, ed 3. St. Louis, Mosby, 1995.

Wasserman, K, Hansen, JE, Sue, DY, and Whipp, BJ: Principles of Exercise Testing and Interpretation. Philadelphia, Lea & Febiger, 1987.

Weiner, DK, Duncan, PW, Chandler, J, and Studenski, SA: Functional reach: a marker of physical frailty. J Am Geriatr Soc 1992, 40:203–207.

Williard, FH: Medical Neuroanatomy. Philadelphia, JB Lippincott, 1993.

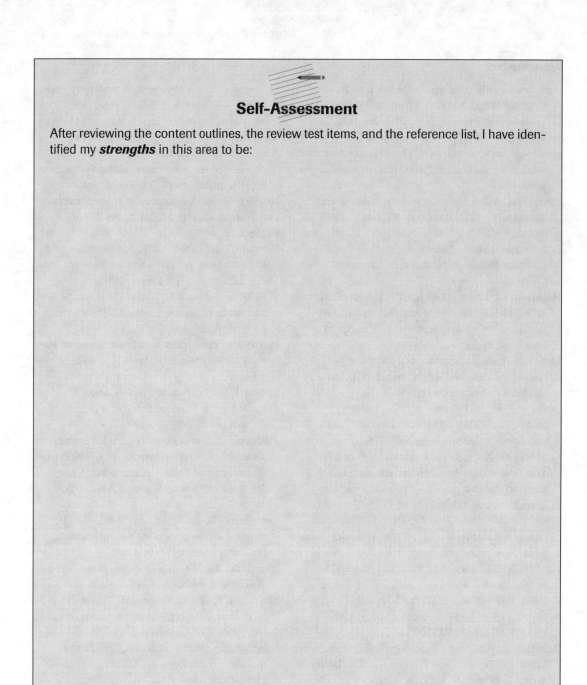

Self-Assessment

After reviewing the content outlines, the review test items, and the reference list, I have identified my *strengths* in this area to be:

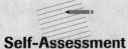

Self-Assessment

After reviewing the content outlines, the review test items, and the reference list, I have identified the following areas in which I need to improve my level of competence:

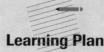

Learning Plan

In order to improve my level of competence, I have identified the following areas of concentrated study, the method(s) by which I will study, and the timelines for each area:

Areas of Concentrated Study:

Learning Plan (Continued):

Methods of Study:

Timelines:

Notes

3 Interpretation and Planning

The second major content area of the examination is Interpretation and Planning, which constitutes 22% of the test items. Thus approximately 44 items on the examination require demonstrated ability to interpret data from evaluation processes, establish a movement dysfunction diagnosis, and plan a treatment regimen that is both effective and efficacious. Within these items are the subcontent areas of data interpretation (13%) and goal setting and care planning (9%). While reviewing this chapter and its respective items, continually ask: What do the data obtained in the subjective and objective evaluations indicate? What do these signs and symptoms represent in the diagnosis of movement dysfunctions? Consider systems and how they function, how they have impact on each other, how to distinguish major from minor problems, and how to prioritize the client's problems.

In the process of delineating a plan of care, select the most appropriate interventions for the client and engage the client in cooperatively established realistic goals. The goals and methods of interventions should reflect an understanding of the impact of socioeconomic and psychosocial factors. It is understood that certain elements of care are delegated to physical therapist assistants and that client and family education are parts of any treatment plan.

As in Chapter 1, competence statements are the primary considerations, with a number of subsets recurring throughout the content outline. Again, this is an indication of the importance of the item or activity and how it transects multiple activities. Following are the subcontent areas identified by the Federation under the rubric of "Interpretation and Planning."

DATA INTERPRETATION

Identify precautions and contraindications to treatment
- Tissue healing times
- Scientific and theoretical basis for various treatments
- Effects of various treatments
- Phases of connective tissue repair and scar tissue formation
- Effects of modalities
- Recognition of allergic reactions to treatment
- Identification of the contraindications for manual therapy
- Signs of life-threatening states (i.e., pulmonary embolus, autonomic dysreflexia)
- Determination if client's signs/symp-

toms are indicative of local and/or systemic origin
- Evaluation of published studies related to physical therapy practice

Determine possible causes of client's problems (i.e., relationships between clients' problems and signs and symptoms)
- How to integrate findings of multiple tests to clarify the client's problem and functional status
- Determination if client's signs/symptoms are indicative of local and/or systemic origin
- Evaluation of published studies related to physical therapy practice

GOAL SETTING AND CARE PLANNING

Select and justify treatments and procedures
- Effects of various treatments
- Rationale for selected treatments
- How to obtain culture specimens by probing tissues with swab, inserting suction catheter into trachea
- Resources that may assist clients and families
- Evaluation of published studies related to physical therapy practice

Establish measurable, short- and long-term goals, and discharge plan for clients in collaboration with patient, family, and health-care team
- How to inform clients regarding the purpose and methods of a procedure, what to expect, and what is expected from them
- Tissue healing times
- Comparison of client response with target response to determine goal achievement
- Determination of whether postural or gait deviations are appropriate adaptations or potentially harmful
- Continuous passive motion (CPM)
- Phases of connective tissue repair and scar tissue formation
- Appropriate professional verbal and written communication skills
- How to record client data in typical measurement units
- Health-care delivery system

Prioritize client problems and associated treatments
- Human anatomy and physiology
- Concepts of human growth and development from conception to senescence, including physical, cognitive, social, and emotional development
- Differentiation of associated causes of dysfunction
- Normal and abnormal findings of assessment procedures
- Identification of normal and abnormal gait

- Rationale for selected treatments
- Health-care delivery system
- Evaluation of published studies related to physical therapy practice
- Critical evaluation of information related to techniques, equipment, and technology related to patient care

Identify appropriate outcome measures
- Purpose of each assessment procedure
- Tissue healing times
- How to write functional goal statements that include activity, standard of performance, limitations allowed, and time frame for achievement
- Effects of various treatments
- Comparison of client response with target response to determine goal achievement
- Health-care delivery system
- Evaluation of published studies related to physical therapy practice

Identify barriers to client progress
- Psychosocial stressors that may affect client response to pain
- How to question client appropriately to assess cognitive status relative to safety, judgment, and reasoning
- Normal and abnormal psychology
- Clinical signs and symptoms of common psychiatric disorders
- Differentiation of associated causes of dysfunction
- Disease processes, indications, contraindications, and precautions for treatment/procedures
- How to alter activities in response to client response
- Underlying impairments that contribute to gait deviations
- Determination if client's signs/symptoms are indicative of local and/or systemic origin
- Resources that may assist clients and families

INTENT OF CONTENT SECTION

The ability to synthesize and interpret data with the goal of establishing a diagnosis of any movement dysfunction regardless of the etiology distinguishes the physical therapist of the late twentieth century from earlier counterparts. The diagnosis rendered by a physical therapist is not a medical diagnosis as in the case of disease; rather, it is a biomechanical and kinesiological evaluation of abnormal movement (i.e., pathokinesiology). From this diagnosis, the physical therapist in partnership with the client is able to establish realistic functional outcome goals and select interventions that offer the highest probability of efficient and effective goal achievement.

As a part of the data-interpretation process, the physical therapist is also obligated to refer the client to another physical therapist or health-care provider when the data indicate that the client's problem is not within the scope, knowledge, or expertise of the therapist conducting the evaluation or within the scope of physical therapy itself. The responsibility to refer is considered one of the basic tenants of professional autonomy. Meticulous attention to the data derived in the evaluation is expected. Recognition of what is or may not be within the scope of physical therapy is an expected characteristic of the contemporary physical therapist.

Foundational work in natural, behavioral, clinical, and other sciences as well as physical therapy science is critical preparation for the practitioner to successfully engage in diagnosis and care-planning activities. Knowledge of contemporary research findings in both the physical therapy literature and related literature enables physical therapists to practice these skills more effectively.

Items that reflect this content area require the test taker to demonstrate knowledge, comprehension, and the ability to apply, analyze, synthesize, and evaluate information. Examples of test items in the content area include:

EXAMPLE #1:

A 60-year-old client is referred for evaluation and treatment planning for left-sided hemiplegia secondary to a cerebrovascular accident (CVA). After the evaluation, it is determined that the client is unable to independently eat or dress, experiences severe shoulder pain during active assistance range of motion, and demonstrates increased tone in both left extremities during ambulation. The primary functional goal for this client will be:

A. unlimited community ambulatory without assistive devices
B. full active range of motion of all four extremities WNL for age and gender
C. pain-free active range of motion of the left upper extremity, particularly glenohumeral motions
D. independence in activities of daily living

The correct response is D. The primary functional goal should be the most inclusive goal. All of the other items include qualifiers that may not be appropriate for this individual. The client may be able to become a community ambulator with assistive devices; however, independence in ambulation is more important than the issue of the assistive devices. Full range of motion may not be possible. It is not known what active range of motion she had before the CVA. Pain-free motion may not be possible and may not inhibit functional independence. Thus, D is the best option in this case.

EXAMPLE #2

The evaluation of a client who sought physical therapy services secondary to increasing shoulder pain while sidelying is complete. Based on the data derived from both the subjective and objective evaluation of this client and knowledge of the literature, it is determined that this type of pain is most commonly due to:

A. too many pillows under the client's head, which causes increased lateral flexion of the neck
B. pressure on the acromion process of the shoulder on which the client is lying
C. pressure on the posterior part of the scapula during sidelying
D. not enough pillows under the client's head, forcing the shoulder to bear more weight

The correct response is B. Analysis of the biomechanical forces on the shoulder joint during sidelying has been identified in the literature as the most common cause of pain. Lateral flexion of the neck after using too many pillows may produce neck pain but not shoulder pain. There is no pressure on the posterior part of the scapula in sidelying, and using insufficient pillows would result in more pressure on the humerus.

SAMPLE TEST ITEMS COVERING INTERPRETATION AND PLANNING CONTENT

Read each item carefully. As in Chapter 1, formulate a correct response. Then look for that response in the choices provided. If the anticipated answer is not among the choices, reread the stem of the item. Then look at each choice separately and determine if the response is true or false. Remember that well-designed items have plausible alternatives. The correct answers are included at the end of the chapter.

1. **A client with an idiopathic spinal "C" curve of more than 60 degrees will probably have a:**

   A. decrease in vital capacity
   B. higher shoulder on the concave side
   C. reluctance to participate in throwing-type sports
   D. posterior rib hump on the concave side

2. **If a client is unable to dorsiflex past neutral, there could be a problem with all of the following except:**

   A. shock absorption at the ankle
   B. ankle rocking
   C. forward progression
   D. stability

3. **The client has a weak tibialis anterior. In what part of the gait cycle would the task of "forward progression" be the most compromised?**

   A. initial contact
   B. terminal stance
   C. pre-swing
   D. initial swing

4. **Restricted shoulder abduction is equal for both active and passive range of motion. Of the following choices, the restriction would most likely be due to:**

   A. deltoid muscle weakness
   B. supraspinatus tendinitis
   C. superior capsule tightness
   D. latissimus dorsi tightness

5. **If a person has a glenohumeral joint capsule tightness restricting external rotation, the best choice of translatoric glide for mobilizing the joint would be:**

   A. superior glide
   B. inferior glide
   C. anterior glide
   D. lateral glide

6. **A 46-year-old gardener presents with left anterior shoulder pain secondary to falling out of a tree and suffering an acromioclavicular sprain. What is expected upon examination?**

   A. full range of motion with end-range pain
   B. pain with movement more than 90 degrees
   C. weakness of the rotator cuff
   D. pain with a PA at 90 degrees

7. **A 50-year-old swimmer presents with left anterior shoulder pain and is unable to initiate the overhead crawl stroke. Pain is described as searing with greatest intensity during external (lateral) rotation. Range of motion is restricted 50% in all movements. These findings are consistent with:**

   A. posterior shoulder instability
   B. acromioclavicular joint arthritis
   C. adhesive capsulitis
   D. impingement

8. **Common areas of pain from glenohumeral dysfunction include all of the following except:**

   A. C5 dermatome
   B. C6 dermatome
   C. deltoid tuberosity
   D. band around the humerus

9. **Clarification about the area of symptoms during forearm supination is necessary because:**

   A. It is very rarely a limited movement.
   B. Supination occurs at both the wrist and elbow.
   C. Clients are generally poor historians.
   D. Supination does not involve the proximal radial-ulnar joint.

10. **A client who had glenohumeral dislocation 6 weeks earlier exhibits weakness and fear reaching up and out beyond 90 degrees of shoulder flexion. The initial goal is to increase glenohumeral stability and patient confidence within the above shoulder level range. Proprioceptive neuromuscular facilitation (PNF) patterns have been chosen for this client. These goals would be best accomplished by beginning with the flexion abduction pattern and:**

    A. working with rhythmic stabilization at and slightly above 90 degrees of flexion
    B. working with traction in the range above 90 degrees
    C. combined isotonics in the range above 90 degrees
    D. passively moving the limb through the full range of motion

11. **A 36-year-old pregnant woman in her third trimester has been referred for evaluation and management. It is determined that she exhibits a diastasis recti (3 fingerwidths wide). Which of the following would be recommended to this client?**

    A. Avoid all abdominal exercises until 6 weeks after giving birth.
    B. Perform abdominal exercises only under the direct supervision of a physical therapist.
    C. Perform abdominal exercises while using your hands to pull the muscle together.
    D. Avoid lifting all objects heavier than 5 lbs.

12. **After evaluating a 38-year-old client, the primary symptom to be addressed is pain over the palmar aspect of the ulnar side of the hand and the fifth digit and the ulnar aspect of the fourth digit. This set of symptoms is probably caused by:**

    A. ulnar nerve irritation at the cubital tunnel
    B. ulnar nerve irritation at the Guyon tunnel
    C. C8 nerve root irritation
    D. all of the above

13. **A 45-year-old client presents with left anterior shoulder pain that increases at night and with overhead activity. He is unable to lie on his left shoulder secondary to pain and cannot abduct his shoulder in the range of 90 to 120 degrees without pain. He notes pain, especially with flexion while his shoulder is internally rotated. Symptoms are consistent with:**

    A. anterior instability
    B. acromioclavicular joint arthritis
    C. impingement syndrome
    D. frozen shoulder

14. **A client reports a decrease in pain with grade II (Maitland scale) manual traction but complains of increased pain with grade III. Based on this finding, the most appropriate treatment technique should be:**

    A. manual traction without tissue stretch
    B. manual traction with tissue stretch short of end range
    C. manual traction with tissue stretch to end of physiological range
    D. mechanical traction to 50% of body weight

15. **A 50-year-old self-referred client seeks evaluation of a movement dysfunction that began 3 months earlier. Chief complaints include generalized fatigue and paraspinal muscle spasms after ambulating 20 ft. She has a long-standing history of gastritis, dysmenorrhea, weight gain of 10 to 15 lbs per year for the past 8 years, and a thyroid condition that fluctuated between hyper- and hypothyroidism. The objective examination reveals long-standing structural scoliosis and no evidence of disk disorder or stenotic changes. The most appropriate course of action is:**

    A. instruction in back stabilization exercise program
    B. referral to the primary care physician
    C. manual and mechanical traction program
    D. referral to a certified orthopedic physical therapist

16. **A 39-year-old high school science teacher complains of left shoulder pain that has lasted for approximately 2 months. The problem began after he played tennis with a cracked racquet. The aggravating factors include reaching back with the left arm, reaching back to put his left arm in his jacket sleeve, and lying on his right side and lifting the bed covers with his left arm. The pain is described as a 3 on a scale of 10 and decreases as soon as the aggravating behavior is stopped. With repetition of activities, the pain increased to a level 5. If both cervical passive accessory intervertebral movements (PAIVMs) (central PAs, C5) and shoulder flexion of 170 degrees produced shoulder or arm pain, the decision should be to:**

    A. recheck shoulder flexion after performing cervical PAIVMs
    B. treat the shoulder and then recheck PAs C5
    C. avoid treating the cervical spine because it may obscure other findings
    D. refer to the primary care physician because there is no evidence of musculoskeletal dysfunction

17. **After reevaluation of a 14-year-old client with a medical diagnosis of Duchenne's muscular dystrophy, it is determined that while he is still ambulatory his energy expenditure requirements increasingly result in less endurance and a greater need for orthotic and assistive devices. This finding:**

    A. is not anticipated at this age
    B. suggests that the client should be referred back to his neurologist
    C. is probably due to obesity
    D. is consistent with skeletal growth for this age

18. **After reviewing the evaluation findings for an 80-year-old client who sustained a closed-head injury in an automobile accident, it is determined that the client is dependent in activities of daily living secondary to left-sided neglect. This is suggestive of injury to the:**

    A. parietal lobe
    B. anterior temporal region
    C. prefrontal area
    D. sensory motor strip

19. **A hold-relax proprioceptive neuromuscular facilitation (PNF) is indicated as part of an exercise program. The literature indicates that hold-relax:**

    A. is synonymous with contract-relax
    B. uses vigorous isometric holds to increase range of motion
    C. uses gentle isometric holds to increase range of motion
    D. is primarily applied to relieve pain and has no effect on range of motion

20. **An isometric contraction anywhere in the range that is followed by an isotonic contract that is done for the purpose of facilitating the agonist and relaxing the antagonist is referred to as:**

    A. repeated contraction
    B. rhythmic initiation
    C. contract relaxation
    D. slow reversal

21. **A client has difficulty stabilizing the right scapula because of weak rhomboids. The PNF pattern of choice to elicit active shortening of the weak muscles would be:**

    A. scapular anterior depression pattern
    B. scapular anterior elevation pattern
    C. D1 extension pattern of the right upper extremity (RUE)
    D. D2 extension pattern of the RUE

22. **When using alternating isometric contractions of the agonist and antagonist muscles in order to stimulate movement of the agonist and to enhance stability at the joint, the techniques are referred to as:**

    A. slow reversal-hold
    B. rhythmic stabilization
    C. approximation
    D. reinforcement

23. **A PNF Diagonal pattern for upper extremity strengthening is indicated for a client who is a hemiplegic secondary to a cerebrovascular accident (CVA). The pattern is the Diagonal Two (D2) pattern identified by Knott and Voss. The patterns of movement will consist of _____ at the glenohumeral joint followed by _____.**

    A. external rotation, adduction, flexion // internal rotation, abduction, extension
    B. internal rotation, abduction, flexion // external rotation, adduction, extension
    C. internal rotation, adduction, flexion // external rotation, abduction, extension
    D. external rotation, abduction, flexion // internal rotation, adduction, extension

24. **Which one of the following exercise programs would be appropriate for an individual with a right thoracic scoliotic curve?**

    A. stretch the right thoracic spine and strengthen the abdominals and gluteals
    B. strengthen the left thoracic spine and stretch the hip flexors and hamstrings
    C. elongate the left side of the thoracic spine and strengthen the right erector spinae
    D. strengthen the left erector spinae to facilitate deep breathing

25. **A 19-year-old client suffered a spinal cord injury. The client was able to demonstrate elbow extension, wrist flexion, and finger extension during manual muscle testing. This would indicate that the level of cord involvement is below:**

    A. C6
    B. C7
    C. C8–T1
    D. T4–T6

26. **A 41-year-old man sought evaluation because of a long-standing neck problem. A right unilateral Gr III mobilization at C4 reproduced the client's symptoms. The client's severity is minimal, irritability is minimal, and stage is chronic. The treatment of choice is:**

    A. left unilateral at C4
    B. manual traction
    C. right rotation at C4
    D. PA at C4

27. **A professional golfer is referred for evaluation and treatment. The referral indicates that the client had an elbow fracture 6 weeks earlier. The client lacks 20 degrees of extension with passive range of motion. Which one of the following techniques is designed to increase extension?**

    A. PA of the radial head on the ulnar
    B. PA of the radial head on the humerus
    C. AP of the coronoid process
    D. distraction of the ulna on the humerus

28. **Distraction is used in peripheral joints for:**

    A. evaluation
    B. pain control
    C. general mobility
    D. all of the above

29. **A 40-year-old client presents with symmetric edema and thickening of the skin of the hands and fingers. These are early signs of:**

    A. scleroderma
    B. systemic lupus erythematosus
    C. osteoarthritis
    D. rheumatoid arthritis

30. **The most common fractures correlated to falls in the elderly include:**

    A. radius, pelvis, and hip
    B. humerus, fibula, and hip
    C. humerus, wrist, pelvis, and hip
    D. pelvis, hip, and tibia

31. **A client presents with a referral for exercise and patient education for a medical diagnosis of ankylosing spondylitis. Which of the following may be an appropriate element of the plan of care?**

    A. instruction in back extension exercises
    B. advice to purchase a soft mattress to allow contour and eliminate pressure points
    C. instruction in back flexion exercises
    D. strengthening exercises for the hip flexors and hamstring musculature

32. **It has been determined that a client should be reevaluated on a weekly basis for the next 30 days. Which part of the overall assessment could a physical therapy aide appropriately perform?**

    A. goniometric measurements
    B. definitive manual muscle testing
    C. gait analysis
    D. none of the above

33. **While evaluating a client with a diagnosis of peripheral neuropathy secondary to alcoholism, it would be appropriate to teach the client's caregiver:**

    A. passive range-of-motion exercises
    B. massage
    C. basic hygiene
    D. all of the above

34. **A physical therapy assistant has recommended that a client be discontinued from further physical therapy. The supervising physical therapist should:**

    A. countersign the recommendation
    B. seek consultation with another physical therapist
    C. reevaluate the client and meet with the physical therapy assistant
    D. discuss the rationale for the recommendation with the physical therapy assistant

35. **A Medicare client with end-stage renal disease has been evaluated. The recommendation is that the client should not receive physical therapy. The rationale is that:**

    A. the client is terminally ill
    B. the client does not demonstrate rehabilitation potential
    C. you believe the client does not want physical therapy services
    D. the client's diagnosis is a contraindication for physical therapy

36. **A colleague seeks consultation about the developmental stage of a child referred for evaluation. The therapist has asked you to consult regarding the evaluation results. The review of the evaluation data indicates the child is unable to reciprocally crawl. This places the child which stage of development?**

    A. 2 months
    B. 4 months
    C. 6 months
    D. 8 months

37. A 36-year-old client was involved in a severe automobile accident and is in an intensive care unit. He is comatose, has right femoral and tibial compound fractures, sternal fractures, right glenohumeral dislocation (reduced), and multiple lacerations of the left extremities and face. He responds to painful stimuli on his left side but not on his right. He demonstrates a positive Babinski sign on the right. There is no reference to either of these last two findings in the chart. The ethical decision at this point is to:

    A. begin passive range of motion of the left extremities
    B. attempt sensory testing on the right
    C. recommend reevaluation in 10 days
    D. contact the primary care physician with your evaluative findings

38. During the evaluation of a 65-year-old retired lumber industry executive who complained of severe pain in the right hip, the following data were obtained: range of motion: right hip flexion of 0 to 110 degrees; abduction of 0 to 20 degrees; lateral rotation of 0 to 45 degrees; and medial rotation of 0 to 5 degrees. Pain is 7 on a scale of 10 while resting and is increased on weight bearing and with movement. The caregiver is instructed in:

    A. manual traction with the hip in slight abduction and lateral rotation
    B. passive range of motion of the hip in pain-free range
    C. mobilization of the hip
    D. resistive range of motion of the hip for all motions

39. A client complains of recurrent moderate to severe headaches after working at a computer for 6 to 8 hours per day. The workstation is evaluated, and it is determined that:

    A. It is ergonomically correct for the client.
    B. The client's problem is the result of self-chosen positioning of materials in the workstation.
    C. The chair height is set too low, causing excessive cervical extension.
    D. The computer desk requires prolonged cervical flexion while the monitor is viewed.

40. A chart review of the physical therapy department is being conducted. After reviewing several charts at random, it is noted that physical therapist X describes all clients with shoulder pain and motion limitations as having adhesive capsulitis. This is questioned because:

    A. The clients are from 50 to 55 years of age.
    B. The gender and ages of the clients are varied.
    C. Most of the clients demonstrate improvement after therapeutic intervention.
    D. All of the clients are referred by the same practitioner.

41. A 48-year-old client is unemployed and does not have health insurance, but the government will pay for physical therapy services. If legally recognized as permanently disabled, which federal program will pay for the services?

    A. Medicare
    B. Medicaid
    C. CHAMPUS
    D. Veteran's Administration

42. **Evaluation findings for a client with recurrent subluxation of the right shoulder will probably lead to an initial exercise program that emphasizes:**

    A. abduction
    B. extension
    C. flexion
    D. medial rotation

43. **A primary short-term functional outcome for a client who had right hip replacement 3 days earlier will be:**

    A. ambulation without assistive devices
    B. independence in bed mobility and transfers
    C. 0 to 10 degrees of hip extension
    D. lateral rotation within normal limits

44. **A client was referred for evaluation and diagnosis of thoracic and lumbar pain. The client reports experiencing nausea in the prone position. This finding suggests:**

    A. herniated lumbar disk
    B. T-9 fracture
    C. facet syndrome T-4
    D. hiatal hernia

45. **A client complains of pain on movement of the left shoulder. Range of motion includes shoulder flexion that is 0 to 180 degrees; lateral rotation is 0 to 90 degrees; medial rotation is 0 to 75 degrees; extension is 0 to 15 degrees; abduction is 0 to 95 degrees; and adduction is 0 to 5 degrees. All of the findings are considered within normal limits except:**

    A. abduction and adduction
    B. flexion and extension
    C. lateral rotation and abduction
    D. medial rotation and abduction

46. **The federally funded program for payment for health-care services for financially indigent persons is:**

    A. Medicare
    B. Medicaid
    C. CHAMPUS
    D. Veteran's Administration

47. **The level of supervision of a physical therapy assistant expected by Medicare is:**

    A. 25%
    B. 50%
    C. 75%
    D. 100%

48. **Which of the following would be considered acceptable in terms of typical measurement units?**

    A. manual muscle testing (MMT): left abductor pollicis brevis 3/5
    B. goniometric measurement of right ankle dorsiflexion: -40 to 30 degrees
    C. MMT: right quadriceps poor to good
    D. goniometric measurement of left index finger: 10 to 60 degrees

49. **The orthotic of choice for a client with a permanent common peroneal nerve injury secondary to a compression injury is:**

    A. AKHFO
    B. KFO
    C. AFO
    D. AO

50. **Medial instability of the knee is evidence of:**

    A. laxity of the medial collateral ligament
    B. a meniscal tear
    C. a fair level of quadriceps strength
    D. a lateral collateral ligamentous tear

51. **Evaluative data reveal anterior and posterior instability of the knee. This is generally an indication of:**

    A. torn medial meniscus
    B. rupture of the lateral collateral ligament
    C. cruciate ligament damage
    D. torn medial collateral ligament

52. **A rapid heart rate is referred to as:**

    A. dysrhythmia
    B. arrhythmia
    C. bradycardia
    D. tachycardia

53. The evaluation of a client with a medical diagnosis of emphysema reveals a consistent impairment that is described as:

    A. restrictive
    B. obstructive
    C. abnormal
    D. pathological

54. Physical therapists are often involved in designing and implementing cardiac rehabilitation programs. Generally these programs are referred to as:

    A. stage I programs
    B. stage II programs
    C. stage III programs
    D. stage IV programs

55. A grocery store checker complained of bilateral wrist and hand pain as well as tingling and numbness. Which of the following is the most likely cause of the condition?

    A. poor posture at the workstation
    B. excessive wrist extension
    C. excessive repetitive wrist flexion
    D. cervical strain injury

56. The brachial plexus tension test results are positive for a client with cervical pain radiating to the RUE. This is indicative of:

    A. nerve root compression
    B. extradural compression
    C. vertebral artery compression
    D. a space-occupying lesion in the cervical spine

57. In an attempt to decrease the space between the head of the humerus and acromion process and elicit pain, a client's upper extremity is forcibly flexed forward. Pain is not elicited; therefore, the _____ is negative.

    A. Adson maneuver
    B. Ludington's test
    C. Yergason's test
    D. impingement sign

58. Unilateral symptoms of pain in the anterior thigh were elicited during the prone knee flexion (Lasegue) test. This is consistent with a _____ nerve root lesion.

    A. C8 or T1
    B. T4 or T5
    C. L2 or L3
    D. S1 or S2

59. In the evaluation of an infant, Barlow's provocative test results were positive. This is an indication of:

    A. hip instability
    B. knee instability
    C. shoulder instability
    D. wrist instability

60. A client presents with paresis of the levator scapulae as well as posterior winging of the inferior portion of the vertebral border of the scapula. The symptoms are consistent with:

    A. direct damage to the dorsal scapular nerve
    B. injury to the C5 nerve root
    C. prolonged stretching injury
    D. damage to the suprascapular nerve

61. A 25-year-old client was referred for weakness of adduction, internal rotation, and external rotation of the hip as well as groin pain that is described as radiating along the medial aspect of the thigh. The physical therapy evaluation confirms that the movement dysfunction is the result of damage to which nerve?

    A. sciatic
    B. femoral
    C. obturator
    D. ilio-inguinal nerve

62. During assessment of a client suspected of having cardiovascular disease, pressure is applied over the carotid sinus. The normal response to this stimulus is:

    A. decrease in the heart rate and a decrease in blood pressure
    B. increase in the heart rate and a decrease in blood pressure
    C. decrease in the heart rate and an increase in blood pressure
    D. increase in the heart rate and an increase in blood pressure

63. Percutaneous electrodes were used in the electrodiagnostic testing of a client. These electrodes record:

    A. multiple motor units
    B. single muscles
    C. single motor unit or just a few motor units
    D. multiple muscle groups

64. Electrodiagnostic testing provided evidence of axonal degeneration distal to injury site. The term used to document this finding is:

    A. axonotmesis
    B. axon response
    C. complex repetitive discharge
    D. contraction fasciculation

65. On the Rancho Los Amigos Cognitive Functioning Scale, a client's ability to engage in goal-directed behavior that is dependent on external direction is documented as level:

    A. II
    B. IV
    C. VI
    D. VIII

66. According to the Braintree Hospital Cognitive Continuum, a client observed as having difficulty initiating attention to purposeful tasks would be at what level?

    A. arousal
    B. low-level attention
    C. attention
    D. low-level organization

67. After the initial evaluation of a client with C4 quadriplegia, functional capabilities are documented as:

    A. totally dependent in activities of daily living
    B. able to feed self without assistive devices
    C. limited self feeding with assistive devices
    D. independent in feeding activities without restriction

68. What is the classification documented for a client with chronic obstructive pulmonary disease who experiences dyspnea during usual activities of daily living but not at rest and can ambulate a mile without dyspnea?

    A. class 1
    B. class 2
    C. class 3
    D. class 4

69. A client sustained burns of both upper extremities. Examination reveals complete destruction of all skin and subcutaneous tissue. This finding is documented as what degree burns?

    A. first
    B. second
    C. third
    D. fourth

70. During a reevaluation of a client with a below-the-knee amputation, residual limb edema is observed. The probable cause identified is:

    A. The client does not wear the prosthesis correctly.
    B. The socket of the prosthesis is too small.
    C. The socket is too far forward.
    D. Quadriceps atrophy is present.

71. **A client with an above-the-knee prosthesis demonstrates excessive knee flexion in early stance. Assessment reveals that the problem is not with the prosthesis. Which of the following is most likely responsible for the excessive knee flexion in early stance?**

    A. weak quadriceps
    B. weak hamstrings
    C. meniscus degeneration
    D. ligamentous instability

72. **A client with an above-the-knee prosthesis demonstrated excessive lateral trunk bending during the swing phase and away from the prosthesis. It is determined that the prosthesis is the cause of the abnormal gait pattern. Which of the following deficits is probably the primary cause of the lateral trunk bending?**

    A. the prosthesis is too long
    B. faulty socket design
    C. excessively high medial wall
    D. inadequate support from posterior brim

73. **A client with a T-5 spinal cord injury has been evaluated. Included in the plan of care is a request for a wheelchair. Which type of wheelchair will most likely be recommended?**

    A. full recliner
    B. semirecliner
    C. active duty lightweight
    D. battery powered

74. **A 14-year-old client with a common peroneal nerve injury has been wearing an ankle fixed orthosis for the past 9 months. The client is unable to stand comfortably. An assessment of the orthosis reveals that the cause of the discomfort is:**

    A. a loose calf band causing a rubbing or friction type irritation over the fibular head
    B. a tight-fitting shoe, especially at the metatarsophalangeal joints
    C. a laxity of the shells, bands, and uprights
    D. an ankle lock is not engaging correctly

75. **A client demonstrated absence of sensation of the face, scalp, eyeball, and tongue. This finding is documented as involvement of which nerve?**

    A. oculomotor
    B. trochlear
    C. trigeminal
    D. facial

76. **During a chart review for a major insurance company, it is noted that the functional outcome of treatment for a client with a cervical root irritation was to increase range of motion, and the treatment provided included ultrasound and massage. Based on this information, it is recommended that:**

    A. the claim be paid
    B. partial payment at a level of 20% of the billable amount be approved
    C. the physical therapist participate in a documentation workshop
    D. the claim as documented be denied

77. **You have determined that your client has a bulging disc at L3 on the left side only. The expected outcome for this client will be:**

    A. increasing trunk flexion range of motion
    B. pain-free activities of daily living
    C. increasing paraspinal muscle strength
    D. elimination of pain

78. **An appropriate functional goal for a 42-year-old client who had a fracture of the right humeral head 12 weeks earlier is to:**

    A. demonstrate 80% range of motion of the right shoulder
    B. achieve good muscle strength level of right shoulder girdle
    C. perform work-related activities pain free with 80% range of motion and strength of the right shoulder
    D. develop compensatory movement patterns to facilitate work related activities

79. **Cervical traction is included in the plan of care for a client with a herniated C5 disc. Which of the following is a true consideration in providing traction for this client?**

    A. Position the client with the neck in 5 degrees of flexion.
    B. Maintain traction for a relatively short period (5 min).
    C. Radicular symptoms should be completely relieved within the first treatment session.
    D. If the symptoms increase, decrease the weight and increase the time.

80. **According to Maitland (Australian approach), the first treatment of choice for a person with right-sided pain and stiffness at C5 is:**

    A. unilateral PA at C5 on the right
    B. manual traction in supine
    C. central PA at C5
    D. rotation to the right at C5

81. **Distraction is used in peripheral joints for:**

    A. evaluation
    B. pain control
    C. general mobility
    D. all of the above

82. **A client's movement dysfunction has been diagnosed as discogenic with nerve root irritation. Based on McKenzie's system of classification, the client has a:**

    A. postural syndrome
    B. dysfunction syndrome
    C. derangement syndrome
    D. degeneration syndrome

83. **Reevaluation of a client reveals that the long-term goals have been achieved. The administrator of the clinical center has issued a directive that all Medicare clients are to remain in the skilled nursing facility for the maximum number of days. This client has only been in the center for 4 days. The most appropriate legal action to be taken is to:**

    A. Determine if the client has any other clinical signs which might warrant physical therapy.
    B. Discharge the client from physical therapy and document achievement of treatment goals.
    C. Comply with the directive from the center administrator.
    D. Indicate in the care plan that the client should be reevaluated in 10 days.

84. **For a 75-year-old client who recently underwent a below-the-knee ambulation secondary to a severe traumatic injury, it is determined that gait training with axillary crutches using a four-point gait pattern is preferable. The rationale for the four-point gait pattern is:**

    A. It will lead to a natural progression to a three-point gait pattern.
    B. It allows the client to learn the most stable gait pattern.
    C. It requires the client to bear weight on the prosthesis.
    D. It means that the weight-bearing status of one extremity must be less than 30% partial weight bearing.

85. **A 68-year-old frail client who lives alone in a one-story home is to be instructed in a touch-down weight-bearing gait pattern. It is decided not to instruct him in the use of:**

    A. axillary crutches
    B. Lofstrand crutches
    C. a pickup walker
    D. a cane

86. Consideration is being given to using cryotherapy as a part of the care plan for a new client. The literature supports the use of cryotherapy for all of the following except:

    A. spasticity
    B. muscle soreness
    C. chronic edema
    D. acute inflammation

87. In acute inflammatory conditions the application of ice has been associated with all of the following except:

    A. reducing edema
    B. raised white blood cell count
    C. reducing spasms
    D. decreasing analgesic intake

88. The client is an experienced equestrian who developed deep, aching pain on the anterior surface of both thighs after a 10-mile ride yesterday. In order to facilitate pain-free gait, what should be included in the plan?

    A. trunk extension exercises
    B. diathermy
    C. pulsed ultrasound
    D. continuous ultrasound

89. Which one of the following is a contraindication for manual stretching?

    A. decreased range of motion because of adhesions
    B. muscle weakness
    C. muscle length imbalance
    D. bony block to joint motion

90. The 38-year-old client was injured in a collision at home plate during a recreational softball game and sustained multiple contusions. Two weeks after the injury, the ecchymosis has resolved and the client can walk without assistive devices. The client continues to report tenderness to touch over the distal quadriceps, pain on weight bearing, and limited knee motion. The evaluation supports these claims. The best soft tissue technique to include in the revised plan of care is:

    A. gentle broadening technique with passive range of motion only
    B. gentle broadening technique with isotonic resistance exercises
    C. gentle lengthening technique with gentle active range-of-motion exercises
    D. gentle lengthening technique with maximal isometric exercises

91. A 20-year-old client is undergoing preseason screening for participation on the college soccer team and demonstrated tight hip flexors. This limitation may makes the client more susceptible to injury. What would be the best technique to increase range of motion of hip extension for this client?

    A. hold-relax through autogenic inhibition of the hip flexors
    B. hold relax through reciprocal inhibition of the hip extensors
    C. ice packs for 15 minutes
    D. effleurage to the hip flexors

92. Closed kinetic chain activities are a part of a care plan. Which one of the following is not an example of a closed kinetic chain activity?

    A. pushup
    B. stairclimber
    C. bench press
    D. lunge

93. A 72-year-old client received a right hip replacement 4 months earlier and 2 weeks earlier experienced a CVA that resulted in left-sided hemiparesis. The client is unable to transfer independently and is unable to ambulate secondary to poor level strength left lower extremity muscle groups. He is also unable to perform activities of daily living (ADLs) involving the left upper extremity secondary to poor level strength all muscle groups. The initial plan of care should include:

    A. PNF techniques for strengthening both upper extremities
    B. L extremities muscle reeducation and gait training
    C. bilateral upper extremity strengthening and ADL training
    D. electrical stimulation left quadriceps and shoulder girdle musculature

94. A 24-year-old client sustained a spinal cord injury as a result of a motorcycle accident. The client has full use of both upper extremities. This is consistent with a level of injury that is below:

    A. C8
    B. T4
    C. T10
    D. L2

95. If a client has had an encapsulated spinal tumor removed, the prognosis is:

    A. grave
    B. poor
    C. fair
    D. excellent

96. Metastatic carcinoma of the breast most commonly occurs in persons who are how old?

    A. 55 to 75 years
    B. 40 to 55 years
    C. 8 to 40 years
    D. 0 to 8 years

97. A client presents with muscle spasms, primarily in the lower extremities but also occurring in the upper extremities, neck, and back. She is 54 years old, postmenopausal, does not take estrogen, and reports no history of any injuries. The onset of symptoms occurred suddenly, and the intensity has remained constant. The decision is to refer her back to her family practitioner. The rationale for the decision is the probability of:

    A. a progressive neurologic disorder
    B. viral infection
    C. an electrolyte imbalance
    D. psychological problem

98. A client is referred for evaluation and management 3 days after injury. The confirmed diagnosis is an ankle sprain with abnormal gait secondary to pain that is markedly increased during push off. The most appropriate first home treatment recommended is:

    A. AAROM within pain-free ROM and ice immersion
    B. AAROM within pain-free ROM, ice, and elevation
    C. AROM within pain-free ROM in whirlpool
    D. PROM within pain-free ROM and ice immersion

99. For the client described in item 98, the caregiver is instructed in taping as a preventive measure. The client is a long-distance runner. In the instructions, the ankle is to be positioned in _____ before taping.

    A. slight dorsiflexion, slight inversion
    B. slight plantarflexion, slight inversion
    C. slight dorsiflexion, slight eversion
    D. slight plantarflexion, slight eversion

100. **The client in the two preceding questions wants to engage in additional progressive treatment. A long-term functional outcome is to return to long-distance running without limitations. Bilateral standing calf raises are a part of the progressive strengthening program. All of the following exercises could be considered progressions in that plan except:**

    A. single leg calf raises
    B. bilateral calf raises off a stair
    C. seated calf raises with heavy-duty 4-inch rubber band
    D. bilateral calf raises on a mini trampoline

101. **A 42-year-old flight attendant sustained a sprained ankle as a result of slipping off a metal stair. Evaluative findings include plantarflexion and eversion: painful and weak; dorsiflexion and eversion: painful and strong. Based on this information, it is determined that there may be some contractile involvement with this sprain. The most likely muscle that injured is the:**

    A. posterior tibialis
    B. anterior tibialis
    C. gastrocnemius
    D. peroneus longus

102. **Another client was referred with an ankle sprain. This 25-year-old client demonstrates abnormal gait because of a lack of great toe extension secondary to severe pain. Manual therapy has been selected to increase great toe extension by using accessory movements. Which of the following is consistent with this plan?**

    A. grade II PA of the phalanx on the metatarsal
    B. grade II AP of the phalanx on the metatarsal
    C. grade IV PA of the phalanx on the metatarsal
    D. grade IV AP of the phalanx on the metatarsal

103. **A 35-year-old client comes to you for evaluation and management of a right medial collateral ligament sprain 18 days ago. After 4 days, the client received a full length leg cast. The cast was removed yesterday. AROM and PROM of the right knee are -10 to 70 degrees. Soft tissue mobilization is included in the plan of care. Which of the following would be the most appropriate for soft tissue mobilization at this time?**

    A. broadening
    B. physiological lengthening
    C. vigorous friction massage
    D. tapotement

104. **For the client in item 103, which one of the following treatments would be most appropriate for decreasing knee pain and chronic swelling?**

    A. hot packs on the right knee for 20 minutes
    B. ultrasound at 1 mHZ, pulsed for 5 minutes to the medial and lateral aspects of the right knee
    C. ice pack for 10 minutes on the right knee
    D. effleurage to the medial and lateral sides of the right knee

105. **For the client in items 103 and 104, quadriceps and hamstrings strength is 4-/5. Which of the following are appropriate in a home exercise program?**

    A. isometric quad sets, 10 repetitions twice a day
    B. squats with 4-inch medium-strength rubber band for resistance in extension, 10 repetitions three times a day
    C. sitting, knee extension against minimal-strength rubber band, 10 repetitions three times a day
    D. prone, active knee flexion, 10 repetitions three times a day

106. **A long-term functional outcome for the client in items 103 to 105 is:**

    A. return to all previous levels of activity 100% painfree
    B. full weight-bearing right lower extremity for 45 minutes without pain
    C. playing racquetball without pain twice a week
    D. no pain, swelling, and full range of motion in the right knee

107. **An active 65-year-old client with a history of arthritis and a fall on concrete pavement complains of severe pain in the left hip, thigh, and low back. Radiographs do not show fractures. Osteoarthritic changes noted. The client reports that sit-to-stand and stepping up or down stairs elicits pain. In the morning, primary symptom is stiffness and pain with hip movement that decreases after 1 or 2 hours. It is concluded that the pain is secondary to contusions, hematoma, and osteoarthritic changes. The client is currently taking prednisone and acetaminophen (Tylenol), which have reduced the pain significantly. An appropriate short-term goal would be:**

    A. pain-free sit-to-stand activities of daily living
    B. walking faster for 25 minutes before onset of pain
    C. increasing right hip AROM to 93 degrees
    D. standing for 20 minutes with pain decreasing after lying down for 30 minutes

108. **For the client in item 107, which one of the following home exercise programs would be most appropriate at this point in time?**

    A. up and down 12 steps three times a day
    B. active ROM of hip flexion, extension, internal rotation, external rotation, abduction, and adduction for 15 minutes three times a day
    C. Tai Chi class for 45 minutes a day
    D. squats, standing on medium strength rubber band to resist hip extension for 20 minutes three times a day

109. **An exercise program is recommended for a 47-year-old person who is 45% over the ideal body weight according to the ameliorization tables. In addition to a diet, which of the following exercise programs would be indicated to assist weight loss?**

    A. jogging for 20 minutes three times a week
    B. riding a stationary bicycle for 20 minutes a day three times a week
    C. slow jogging for 30 minutes four times a week
    D. slow walking for 40 minutes four times a week

110. **The client is an 80-year-old Asian Pacific Islander who speaks limited English. Her primary language is Mandarin Chinese. One of the major considerations in the planning process is:**

    A. accomplishing the established goals in the most expeditious manner
    B. involving other health-care providers in her care
    C. respecting cultural mores regarding touching
    D. identifying the payor for her services and the limitations imposed on care

111. **The rationale for utilizing Brunnstrom's rowing technique of alternating flexion and extension in and out of synergy is that it is a technique:**

    A. for isolating the arms with a goal of increasing separation from the trunk
    B. for promoting movement in patients who have just begun volitional movement of the biceps and triceps
    C. primarily used to promote bilateral upper extremity and trunk ROM
    D. that attempts to achieve overflow from the uninvolved side to help coordinate alternating movements of the involved side

112. **In accordance with Brunnstrom's treatment theory, when a client with a CVA demonstrates synergy patterns:**

    A. encourage the client to stay out of the synergy pattern
    B. it means nothing; Brunnstrom says nothing about such patterns
    C. use the strong components of the synergy to facilitate activation of weaker muscles
    D. have the client bear weight through the extremity to normalize tone

113. **A 24-year-old client who suffered a left CVA-like trauma secondary to a mycotic bacterium–related middle cerebral artery hemorrhage has recovered significant functional ability; however, he has difficulty in extending his right hip during the stance phase. The decision is to use PNF as part of the plan of care. Which of the following positions and techniques would be best to try at this point in time?**

    A. quadruped using slow reversals in a D1 extension pattern
    B. half kneeling on right lower extremity, rhythmic stabilization, resisting right extension in a diagonal while applying slight abduction resistance on the left lower extremity
    C. sidelying on elbows using combined isotonics in a D1 extension pattern
    D. supine RI in a bilateral symmetrical left extremity flexion pattern

114. **A 26-year-old obese client complains of central lumbar pain radiating down the back of the right thigh and leg to the heel. Pain began suddenly after the client reached down to pick up a book, and it is aggravated by sitting and lying on the right and eased by standing and walking. Which one of the following traction techniques is initially appropriate?**

    A. supine, intermittent mechanical traction of 45 lbs for 20 minutes
    B. prone, continuous traction of 45 lbs
    C. supine, sustained traction of 70 lbs for 10 minutes
    D. prone, manual traction for 1 to 2 minutes

115. **In establishing a home care plan for a Medicaid client, one of the major considerations should be:**

    A. efficacy of the treatment proposed
    B. cost to the client
    C. relationship to full recovery
    D. reimbursable components

116. On reevaluation, it is decided to apply neurodevelopmental techniques (NDTs) to progress a client's treatment. Which of the following is not a NDT principle for progression?

    A. gait training straight ahead before practicing turning around
    B. focusing on refining distal skills to increase stability proximally
    C. performing reciprocal knee bends in parallel stance before stepping forward and back
    D. occasionally attempting higher-level skills to improve the patient's ability to perform lower-level skills

117. The postural support components of a wheelchair seating system include:

    A. seat and back
    B. head support
    C. anterior chest strap
    D. all of the above

118. Back height is an important consideration in fitting a client's wheelchair. A client with quadriplegia who will be pushing the wheelchair independently requires a back height that is:

    A. at the level of the midpoint of the scapula, for proper support and stability
    B. just above the level of the postero-superior iliac spine
    C. below the inferior angle of the scapula
    D. at the top of the shoulder for best trunk support

119. Wheelchairs for sports are:

    A. more likely to be reimbursable when billed as "high mobility" use rather than for sport activities
    B. constructed of heavy steel frames for increased sturdiness
    C. equipped with smooth, narrow tires for off-road, multiterrain activities
    D. not appropriate for individuals over 50 years of age

120. The client has a spinal cord injury, L1, 3 months post injury. Starting a week ago, the client describes his desire to walk by the next holiday. It is learned that a nurse's aide (CNA) has been encouraging the client not to give up hope of "walking home." What is the most appropriate action?

    A. Encourage the client to keep thinking positive and remain ambiguous about walking.
    B. Speak to the CNA about the client's realistic chances for recovery, and set up goals for the client to accomplish before attempting to ambulate.
    C. Refer the client to a stress counselor or clinical psychologist for evaluation and counseling.
    D. Ignore the questions about walking and speak to the director of nursing about the aide.

121. The highest level of spinal cord injury at which it is possible for a client to be independent with transfers is:

    A. C5
    B. C6
    C. C7
    D. T1

122. The following are all generally part of the management of a client with lumbar spinal cord injury in the subacute stage except:

    A. resistive exercises for strength training of retained muscles
    B. cardiovascular training
    C. wheelchair mobility training, including performing wheelies
    D. respiratory techniques, including percussion and vibration

123. In the acute phase after cervical or thoracic spinal cord injury, all of the following could be appropriate interventions after a client receives orthopedic clearance except:

A. acclimation to vertical
B. achievement of full passive range of motion in all joints
C. selective strengthening
D. assisted respiration techniques

124. Biofeedback used in combination with relaxation therapy:

A. must only be performed by a person who is trained in clinical psychology
B. is effective because it refocuses the client's attention
C. is particularly beneficial for clients who find it difficult to relax or those with stress-related disorders
D. is more useful for clients believed to have a psychological component contributing to their dysfunction

125. The main problems you identify for a 70-year-old man with Parkinson's disease would include all of the following except:

A. decreased balance
B. bradykinesia
C. kyphotic posture
D. hypotonicity

126. The most appropriate sequence of activities to be used in gait training progression from easier to harder tasks is:

A. lateral weight shift; single leg stance; diagonal weight shift; side stepping
B. lateral weight shift; diagonal weight shift; single leg stance; braiding
C. stride weight shifts; lateral weight shifts; side step; single leg stance
D. lateral weight shifts; single leg stance; side stepping; hip hiking

127. In planning an intervention for an agitated head-injured client, a major consideration is:

A. to continually verbalize reassurances of the safety of what you are doing
B. to touch the client to calm him
C. to use simple, one-step commands and speak in short, simple sentences
D. to speak and touch firmly throughout the treatment session

128. One of the cardinal rules of skin care in which the physical therapist should educate the client and the caregivers is to:

A. change positions every 4 hours while in bed
B. remove cushions from chairs
C. avoid friction on body parts during transfers
D. wear comparatively tight-fitting clothing for support

129. In managing a client referred for dizziness, the treatment will involve challenging the vestibular system:

A. without causing dizziness with emphasis on incorporating as many different positions as time allows
B. with emphasis on achieving the maximum amount of dizziness and holding the positions that elicit dizziness for 5 to 7 minutes or until dizziness subsides
C. with emphasis on merely eliciting dizziness and having the client maintain the position for as long as necessary to relieve all dizziness
D. facilitating movements that elicit moderate dizziness and having the client maintain these positions for 10 to 15 seconds if dizziness does not diminish

130. Appropriate written documentation to a referring physician rather than a third-party payor or a caregiver includes:

A. remaining positive in spite of the severity of the diagnosis
B. providing succinct problem statements, goals, and plans
C. giving only functional information indicating the level of dependency of the client
D. suggestions for pharmaceutical changes that will improve the client's function

131. The source of deep somatic pain is:

A. superficial somatic structures
B. bone, nerve, muscle, or tendon
C. organs of respiration and digestion
D. any of the above

132. If a client indicates that the pain intensifies or builds up with movement and subsides with rest, it is consistent with:

A. irritation
B. inflammation
C. ischemia
D. infection

133. The source of the pain for the client described in the previous question is:

A. superficial somatic structures
B. bone, nerve, muscle, or tendon
C. organs of respiration, digestion, urogenital
D. any of the above

134. Clients whose pain increases with systolic pressure (e.g., exercise or bending over) are referred to as having what kind of pain?

A. arterial
B. pleural
C. tracheal
D. heart

135. A client demonstrates trunk flexion and tilts toward the painful side in order to compensate for pain. In addition to a musculoskeletal dysfunction what may be the cause of this postural pattern?

A. pancreatic pain
B. swollen kidney
C. distended gallbladder
D. gastritis

136. A hyperirritable spot within a tight band of muscle is:

A. a fibrous nodule
B. excessive calcium
C. referred pain
D. a trigger point

137. The five "P's"—pain, pallor, pulselessness, paresthesia, and paralysis—are indicative of:

A. cerebrovascular hemorrhage
B. psychosomatic dysfunctions
C. acute arterial occlusion
D. nerve root irritations

138. The pain associated with _____ _____ is often very deep, aching, and throbbing. Pressure may reduce this type of pain.

A. systemic joint disease
B. spinal stenosis
C. symptom magnification syndrome
D. posttraumatic hyperirritability syndrome

139. A 40-year-old woman client who is 5 months' pregnant experiences increased Braxton Hicks contractions during exercise. This is indicative of:

A. a need for more frequent rest intervals
B. decreased calcium and potassium levels
C. a need for medical attention
D. a systemic problem

140. Which of the following is a contraindication to physical therapy intervention?

A. resting heart rate of 82 BPM
B. resting systolic rate of 190 mm Hg
C. resting diastolic rate of 95 mm Hg
D. fatigue

141. A client with diabetes demonstrates marked confusion and lethargy during the evaluation session. The appropriate action to take is to:

A. give the client orange juice
B. call 911
C. contact the caregiver
D. call the primary care physician

142. If a therapist is unable to reproduce a female client's back and hip pain, it is appropriate to:

A. implement a simple, nonstrenuous exercise program
B. refer the client to a physical therapist specializing in women's health
C. ascertain how recently the client has been evaluated by a gynecologist and refer if indicated
D. proceed with establishing a plan of care and implement it for three to six visits

143. In the interview of a male client who reports sacroiliac pain, it is important to:

A. determine whether urogenital problems may also exist
B. ensure that the treating therapist is also a man
C. distinguish clearly between prostate and musculoskeletal conditions
D. seek validation of findings by a primary care physician

144. The rationale for women to receive hormone replacement therapy is that:

A. The risk of early development of symptomatic cerebrovascular disease is greater in women than in men.
B. There is a higher incidence of survival with uterine cancer.
C. It decreases the incidence of peripheral neuropathies in later years.
D. Estrogen increases high-density lipoprotein (HDL) levels and thus acts as a protection factor.

145. Cholesterol levels of 240mg/dL with ratios of total cholesterol to HDL of more than 4.0 result in:

A. obesity that is extremely difficult to manage
B. twice as high a risk for heart disease
C. decreased exercise capacity
D. the same risk of heart disease as a smoker

146. Percutaneous transluminal coronary angioplasty (PTCA) is used to:

A. compress the plaque in an artery, thus halting the progressiveness of coronary artery disease (CAD)
B. bypass diseased vessels and create increased blood flow
C. ease the symptoms of a blocked coronary artery
D. predict the onset of CAD

147. A client who complains of pain behind the sternum that radiates to the jaw is probably describing:

A. angina pectoris
B. heartburn
C. myocardial ischemia
D. vascular claudication

148. **Pitting edema, paroxysmal dyspnea, dizziness, and syncope are clinical signs and symptoms of:**

    A. an aneurysm
    B. cardiac valvular disease
    C. right ventricular failure
    D. pericarditis

149. **A physical therapist is working with a client who recently had a stroke. When checking the client's pulse, it is critical to monitor for:**

    A. bradycardia
    B. tachycardia
    C. fibrillations
    D. dysrhythmias

150. **Raynaud's disease is a primary vasospastic disorder. The cause of the disease is:**

    A. hypersensitivity of digital arteries to cold
    B. release of serotonin
    C. a congenital predisposition
    D. any of the above

151. **While reevaluating a client who underwent a knee replacement the following differences are observed: sudden difficulty in speaking, blindness, and decreased strength in the left extremities. These clinical signs and symptoms are consistent with:**

    A. post-anesthesia recovery
    B. a transient ischemic attack
    C. an allergic reaction to one or more medications
    D. hypertension

152. **An elderly client complains of a sense of weakness or "rubbery" legs, visual blurring, and lightheadedness as well as syncope. These are clinical signs and symptoms of:**

    A. orthostatic hypotension
    B. a pulmonary embolism
    C. chronic hypertension
    D. a transient ischemic attack

153. **Superficial lateral or anterior chest wall pain that is aggravated by exertion of only the upper body and follows a history of back pain is indicative of:**

    A. herpes zoster
    B. thoracic outlet syndrome
    C. dorsal nerve root irritation
    D. anxiety state/panic disorder

154. **Compression of the neural and vascular structures that leave or pass over the superior rim of the thoracic cage describes:**

    A. herpes zoster
    B. thoracic outlet syndrome
    C. dorsal nerve root irritation
    D. anxiety state or panic disorder

155. **The pain pattern associated with pericarditis is substernal and:**

    A. radiates to the medial aspects of both upper extremities, the left more frequently than right
    B. projects to the left shoulder and arm over the distribution of the ulnar nerve
    C. radiates to the neck, interscapular area, shoulders, lower back, or abdomen
    D. radiates anteriorly to the costal margins, neck, upper back, upper trapezius, and left supraclavicular area or down the left arm

156. **A common pain pattern associated with myocardial infarctions is substernal and:**

    A. radiates to the medial aspects of both upper extremities, the left more frequently than right
    B. projects to the left shoulder and arm over the distribution of the ulnar nerve
    C. radiates to the neck, interscapular area, shoulders, lower back, or abdomen
    D. radiates anteriorly to the costal margins, neck, upper back, upper trapezius, and left supraclavicular area or down the left arm

157. A client who has been diagnosed as having angina will report pain that is substernal and:

A. radiates to the medial aspects of both upper extremities, the left more frequently than right

B. projects to the left shoulder and arm over the distribution of the ulnar nerve

C. radiates to the neck, interscapular area, shoulders, lower back, or abdomen

D. radiates anteriorly to the costal margins, neck, upper back, upper trapezius, and left supraclavicular area or down the left arm

158. Clients with dissecting aortic aneurysms present with pain that:

A. radiates to the medial aspects of both upper extremities, the left more frequently than right

B. projects to the left shoulder and arm over the distribution of the ulnar nerve

C. radiates to the neck, interscapular area, shoulders, lower back, or abdomen

D. radiates anteriorly to the costal margins, neck, upper back, upper trapezius, and left supraclavicular area or down the left arm

159. If a client reports anginal pain that is not relieved in 20 minutes, the most appropriate action to be taken by the physical therapist is:

A. cessation of the evaluation or treatment session

B. positioning the client supine with the feet elevated above the heart

C. dependent on the client's history and current medications

D. immediately seek medical attention for the client

160. A client who wakes up at night gasping for air has:

A. dyspnea

B. paroxysmal nocturnal dyspnea

C. valvular insufficiency

D. hypertension

161. Any condition that decreases pulmonary ventilation and increases retention and concentration of CO_2, hydrogen, and carbonic acid is called:

A. respiratory acidosis

B. respiratory alkalosis

C. chronic obstructive pulmonary disease

D. asthma

162. If a client's condition results in bronchial dilation with inflammation, the disease is:

A. bronchitis

B. bronchiectasis

C. pneumonia

D. cystic fibrosis

163. A disease that is characterized by obstruction and obliteration of the bronchioles is:

A. bronchitis

B. bronchiectasis

C. pneumonia

D. cystic fibrosis

164. Increased respiratory rate, pursed-lip breathing, and use of accessory muscles for respiration are consistent signs and symptoms of:

A. emphysema

B. asthma

C. pneumonia

D. tuberculosis

165. Major clinical symptoms of brain metastasis are:

A. chest, shoulder, or arm pain

B. bowel and bladder incontinence, diminished or absent extremity reflexes

C. headache, weakness, and malaise

D. atrophy and weakness of the extremities, either unilaterally or bilaterally

166. **A client with hemophilia sustained a knee injury. The client demonstrates gradually intensifying pain, protective spasm of the quadriceps, loss of range of motion, and loss of sensation in the knee area. These signs and symptoms are consistent with:**

    A. acute hemarthrosis
    B. thrombocytopenia
    C. muscle hemorrhage
    D. leukocytosis

167. **A client was injured in a soccer game when forcibly tackled from the right and had the "wind knocked out" of him. The client finished the game after a 20-minute rest, but awoke the next morning with severe left shoulder pain. A few hours later the client stopped by a physical therapist's office. Upon evaluation, no loss of motion was discovered despite the client's complaint of "constant pain." The physical therapist referred the client to a primary care physician immediately, suspecting:**

    A. subluxation of the shoulder with immediate resolution
    B. a vertebral fracture at C-7
    C. a ruptured spleen
    D. hemorrhaging within the shoulder

168. **A client was referred for evaluation of radiating back pain. During the interview the symptoms and signs were identified: epigastric pain 45 to 60 minutes after meals that is relieved by food, milk, or antacids; night pain (12 midnight to 3:00 AM); weight loss; bloody stools; occasional right shoulder pain; and radiating back pain. These signs and symptoms are consistent with:**

    A. a peptic ulcer
    B. degenerative disk disease
    C. facet syndrome at T-4
    D. Crohn's disease

169. **As a part of the evaluation of a person with unilateral lumbar pain, the client is prone and the therapist places one hand over the twelfth rib at the costovertebral angle on the back. The other hand is used to "thump" the hand resting on the back. If the client reports no pain, merely a thud, the therapist may rule out:**

    A. lumbar disk impairment
    B. a nerve root irritation
    C. kidney involvement
    D. protective muscle spasms

170. **A common condition observed in clients with acromegaly is:**

    A. arthralgias
    B. progressive fatigue that responds to rest
    C. muscle cramping
    D. carpal tunnel syndrome

171. **A client referred for evaluation of arthritic type symptoms has a history of Cushing's syndrome. Externally applied corticosteroids are a possible treatment. A rationale for not using corticosteroids is:**

    A. the increase in serum cortisol levels triggers a negative feedback signal to the anterior pituitary gland to stop secreting adrenocorticotropic hormone (ACTH)
    B. it may result in adrenal insufficiency with resulting decreased production of cortisol and aldosterone
    C. that an excess of vasopressin may result leading to marked water retention
    D. the thyroid-stimulating hormone (TSH) level will be excessively high

172. Proximal muscle weakness is common in clients who have _____ _____ as are complaints of aches, pains, cramps, and stiffness. Persistent myofascial trigger points are also present. Any compromise of the client's energy metabolism of muscle aggravates and increases the trigger points.

    A. hypothyroidism
    B. hyperparathyroidism
    C. diabetes mellitus
    D. periarthritis

173. A condition commonly associated with diabetes mellitus that is believed to be related to fibroblast proliferation in the connective tissue structures is:

    A. adhesive capsulitis
    B. tendinitis
    C. myositis
    D. periarthritis

174. Diabetic neuropathies commonly referred to as carpal tunnel syndromes are thought to be the result of:

    A. microtrauma to the radial nerves secondary to infection
    B. repetitive use activities
    C. ischemia of the median nerve secondary to microvascular damage
    D. erratic insulin action related to irregular dietary, exercise, and rest habits

175. Clients requiring insulin by injection rarely use intramuscular sites because:

    A. intravenous sites are easier to use
    B. of inconsistent absorption rates
    C. of difficulty in technique
    D. fatty subcutaneous tissue does not have a good absorption rate

176. The most significant side effect of insulin therapy is:

    A. hypoglycemia
    B. lipodystrophy
    C. an allergic reaction
    D. progressive accommodation

177. After preseason screening of a high school football player who demonstrated poor motor coordination, decreased mental alertness, and sudden weight gain with mild peripheral edema, the physical therapist refers the athlete to the team physician. The therapist suspected:

    A. diabetes mellitus
    B. dehydration
    C. water intoxication
    D. hypoglycemia

178. An elderly client suffered a compression fracture of a thoracic vertebra. During the evaluation the client also acknowledged a 1.5-inch decrease in height during the past 3 years and previous low thoracic and upper lumbar pain. It is noted that the client is markedly kyphotic and exhibits a Dowager's hump. These findings are consistent with a diagnosis of:

    A. osteoporosis
    B. osteomalacia
    C. gout
    D. hemochromatosis

179. A long-term viral disease that results in bone becoming spongelike, weakened, and deformed is:

    A. osteogenesis imperfecta
    B. Paget's disease
    C. ochronosis
    D. primary gout

180. The inherited condition that is transmitted by an autosomal dominant gene and is an abnormality in collagen synthesis that leads to increased bone fragility is:

    A. osteoporosis
    B. ochronosis
    C. Paget's disease
    D. osteogenesis imperfecta

181. There are two types of malignant tumors. The type that consists of a large percentage of dividing cells with many abnormal chromosomes is referred to as:

    A. metastatic
    B. benign
    C. invasive
    D. none of the above

182. Malignant tumors that develop from connective tissues are known as:

    A. carcinomas
    B. sarcomas
    C. lymphomas
    D. leukemias

183. Tumors that arise from epithelial cells and metastasize via the lymphatics are referred to as:

    A. carcinomas
    B. sarcomas
    C. lymphomas
    D. leukemias

184. Neuroblastomas are common in which age group?

    A. 0 to 8 years
    B. 8 to 40 years
    C. 40 to 55 years
    D. 55 to 75 years

185. Secondary osteogenic sarcomas are common in which age group?

    A. 0 to 8 years
    B. 8 to 40 years
    C. 40 to 55 years
    D. 55 to 75 years

186. Metastatic carcinoma of the breast and prostate are most commonly found in which age group?

    A. 0 to 8 years
    B. 8 to 40 years
    C. 40 to 55 years
    D. 55 to 75 years

187. Primary tumors of the central nervous system _____ develop metastases outside the central nervous system (CNS).

    A. never
    B. rarely
    C. frequently
    D. always

188. Which of the following is a biologic mechanism in the development of chronic cancer pain?

    A. bone destruction
    B. obstruction
    C. distention
    D. all of the above

189. A 70-year-old client was evaluated for loss of functional left shoulder motion. Evaluation revealed mild loss of strength in the left upper extremity (LUE) with mild sensory and proprioceptive losses. Palpation of the shoulder elicited breast pain. There were positive trigger points of the left pectoralis major and minor as well as a loss of accessory motions of the left shoulder. The client reported having suffered a stroke 10 years earlier. The physical therapist has decided to implement treatment for one week. The goals of the treatment are to:

    A. restore shoulder motion and eliminate trigger points in order to achieve pain-free performance of activities of daily living
    B. restore cervical and shoulder range of motion as well as to strengthen the LUE
    C. alleviate pain before initiating a strengthening program
    D. promote sensory and proprioceptive integrity in order to perform activities of daily living independently

190. During an evaluation of a 35-year-old client who complains of pain radiating from the neck to the left shoulder, the physical therapist palpated a lymph node that measured 2.5 cm. and was firm to touch. The client reported experiencing night sweats, weight loss, edema, and fatigue. The physical therapist decided not to proceed with any treatment and referred the client to a primary care physician. The client's symptoms and the therapist's findings are consistent with:

    A. multiple myelomas
    B. non-Hodgkin's lymphoma
    C. Hodgkin's disease
    D. soft tissue sarcomas

191. Osteosarcomas are the most common type of bone cancer, occurring most commonly in boys aged 10 to 25 years. This usual site for this type of cancer is:

    A. pelvic bones
    B. epiphyses of long bones
    C. tibia and fibula
    D. vertebrae

192. A 45-year-old client who underwent a hemipelvectomy secondary to metastatic cancer was evaluated to determine rehabilitation potential. The client has been otherwise healthy. Strength in remaining extremities is 5/5. Endurance is limited secondary to bedrest. Based only on the type of amputation, the client's potential for ambulation is:

    A. good with prosthesis and crutches
    B. good for independent ambulation with prosthesis alone
    C. fair and will depend on motivation
    D. nonexistent; the client will not ambulate

193. A primary tumor of the central nervous system (CNS) that is within the spinal cord is referred to as:

    A. intradural
    B. extradural
    C. extramedullary
    D. intramedullary

194. More than 80 percent of CNS tumors occur:

    A. extracranial
    B. intramedullary
    C. intracranially
    D. extramedullary

195. A client being evaluated received an organ transplant from an identical twin. This type of transplants is referred to as:

    A. allogeneic
    B. syngeneic
    C. autologous
    D. xenogeneic

196. The use of an animal organ for transplant to a human is referred to as:

    A. allogeneic
    B. syngeneic
    C. autologous
    D. xenogeneic

197. Which group of neurological disorders has an immunologic basis in which the autoimmune mechanisms cause a block or destruction of the acetylcholine receptor lying within the postsynaptic muscle membrane

    A. myasthenia gravis
    B. Guillain-Barré syndrome
    C. multiple sclerosis
    D. muscular dystrophy

198. **A chronic, systemic, inflammatory disorder of unknown etiology that can affect various organs but predominantly involves the synovial tissues of the diarthrodial joints is:**

    A. Sjögren's syndrome
    B. rheumatoid arthritis
    C. systemic lupus erythematosus
    D. scleroderma

199. **A 34-year-old client presents with thoracolumbar pain and stiffness of 5 months duration. Pain is usually worse in the morning, is achy and sometimes sharp, and resolves in about 1 hour. The onset was insidious. Paravertebral muscle spasms occur frequently, and there seems to be a slow progressive limiting of motion. Decreased mobility is symmetrical in the anteroposterior and lateral planes. These symptoms are consistent with:**

    A. Reiter's syndrome
    B. polymyositis
    C. ankylosing spondylitis
    D. fibromyalgia

200. **When comparing systemic and musculoskeletal joint pain, which of the following is consistent with a systemic cause?**

    A. pain is sharp
    B. the client awakens at night
    C. pain decreases with rest
    D. trigger points are accompanied by nausea and sweating

Correct Responses to Sample Items in Chapter 3

The following are the correct responses to items 1 to 200 contained in this chapter.

1. A	51. C	101. D	151. B
2. B	52. D	102. D	152. A
3. C	53. B	103. B	153. C
4. C	54. B	104. A	154. B
5. A	55. C	105. C	155. D
6. B	56. A	106. A	156. A
7. C	57. D	107. A	157. B
8. B	58. C	108. B	158. C
9. B	59. A	109. A	159. D
10. A	60. B	110. C	160. B
11. C	61. C	111. D	161. A
12. B	62. A	112. C	162. B
13. C	63. C	113. B	163. D
14. B	64. A	114. A	164. A
15. B	65. C	115. B	165. C
16. A	66. A	116. B	166. C
17. D	67. C	117. D	167. B
18. C	68. C	118. C	168. A
19. C	69. D	119. A	169. C
20. A	70. B	120. B	170. D
21. C	71. A	121. B	171. B
22. B	72. C	122. D	172. A
23. D	73. A	123. B	173. D
24. C	74. B	124. C	174. C
25. B	75. C	125. D	175. B
26. A	76. D	126. B	176. A
27. D	77. B	127. C	177. C
28. D	78. C	128. C	178. A
29. A	79. B	129. D	179. B
30. C	80. A	130. B	180. D
31. A	81. D	131. B	181. C
32. A	82. C	132. C	182. B
33. D	83. B	133. D	183. A
34. C	84. B	134. A	184. A
35. B	85. D	135. B	185. D
36. B	86. C	136. D	186. D
37. D	87. B	137. C	187. B
38. A	88. A	138. A	188. D
39. C	89. D	139. C	189. A
40. B	90. C	140. B	190. C
41. A	91. A	141. B	191. B
42. D	92. C	142. C	192. A
43. B	93. B	143. A	193. D
44. C	94. A	144. D	194. C
45. A	95. D	145. B	195. B
46. B	96. A	146. C	196. D
47. B	97. C	147. A	197. A
48. A	98. B	148. B	198. B
49. C	99. C	149. D	199. C
50. A	100. C	150. D	200. B

References:

All of the references identified in Chapter 2 were also used in the development of sample test items for this chapter. In addition, the following references were used:

Bailey, DM: Research for the Health Professional: A Practical Guide, ed 2. Philadelphia, FA Davis, 1997.

Barnes, ML, and Scully, R: Physical Therapy. Philadelphia, WB Saunders, 1990.

Bodenheimer, RS, and Grumbach, K: Understanding Health Policy: A Clinical Approach. Norwalk, CT, Appleton & Lange, 1995.

Boyling, JD, and Palastanga, N: Grieve's Modern Manual Therapy, ed 2. New York, Churchill-Livingstone, 1994.

Brodal, A: Neurological Anatomy, ed 3. London, Oxford University Press, 1981.

Brooks, VB: The Neural Basis of Motor Control. London, Oxford University Press, 1986.

Bullock, BL: Pathophysiology: Adaptations and Alterations in Function, ed 4. Philadelphia, JB Lippincott, 1996.

Cyriax, J: Fundamentals of Orthopaedics. Philadelphia, WB Saunders, 1984.

Electrotherapy Standards Committee of the Section on Clinical Electrophysiology: Electrotherapeutic Terminology in Physical Therapy. Alexandria, VA, American Physical Therapy Association, 1990.

Enwemeka, CS: Laser biostimulation of healing wounds: Specific effects and mechanisms of action. J Ortho Sport Phys Ther 1988:9:333–338.

Fischbach, FT: A Manual of Laboratory and Diagnostic Tests, ed 4. Philadelphia, JB Lippincott, 1992.

Gilman, S, and Winans-Newman, S: Manter and Gatz's Essentials of Clinical Neuroanatomy and Neurophysiology, ed 8. Philadelphia, FA Davis, 1992.

Goodman, CC, and Snyder, TEK: Differential Diagnosis in Physical Therapy, ed 2. Philadelphia, WB Saunders, 1995.

Held, JM: In Cohen, H.: Neuroscience for Rehabilitation. Philadelphia, JB Lippincott, 1993.

Horak, FB: Assumptions Underlying Motor Control for Neurologic Rehabilitation. In Contemporary Management of Motor Control Problems: Proceedings of the II Step Conference. Alexandria, VA, Foundation for Physical Therapy, 1991.

Horak, FB, and Nashner, LM: Central programming of postural movements: Adaptations to altered support-surface configurations. J Neurophys 1986, 55:1369–1381.

Kaplan, PE, and Tanner, ED: Musculoskeletal Pain and Disability. Norwalk, CT, Appleton & Lange, 1989.

Kerlinger, FN: Behavioral Research: A Conceptual Approach. San Francisco, Holt, Rinehart and Winston, 1979.

Kiernan, JA: Introduction to Human Neuroscience. Philadelphia, JB Lippincott, 1987.

Fletcher, GF: Rehabilitation Medicine: Contemporary Clinical Perspectives. Baltimore, Williams & Wilkins, 1992.

The Merck Manual of Diagnosis and Therapy, ed. 16. Rahway, NJ, Merck, 1992.

Michlovitz, S: Thermal Agents in Rehabilitation. Philadelphia, FA Davis, 1996.

Monahan, B: Managing Under Managed Care. Physical Therapy Magazine 1994, 4:34–40.

Murphy, GP, Lawrence, WL, and Lenhard, E: American Cancer Society Textbook of Clinical Oncology. Washington, DC, American Cancer Society, 1995.

Observational Gait Analysis: Downey, CA, Rancho Los Amigos Medical Center, 1993.

Payton, OD: Research: The Validation of Clinical Practice, ed 3. Philadelphia, FA Davis, 1994.

Portney, L, and Watkins, M: Foundations of Clinical Research, Applications to Practice. East Norwalk, CT, Appleton & Lange, 1993.

Saunders, HD, and Saunders, R: Evaluation, Treatment and Prevention of Musculoskeletal Disorders, vol 1. Edina, MN, Educational Opportunities, 1994.

Snyder, ML, and Robinson, AJ: Clinical Electrophysiology: Electrotherapy and Electrophysiologic Testing. Baltimore, Williams & Wilkins, 1995.

Tomberlin, JP, and Saunders, HD: Evaluation, Treatment and Prevention of Musculoskeletal Disorders, vol 2. Edina, MN, Educational Opportunities, 1994.

Schumway-Cook, A, and Woolcott, MH: Motor Control Theory and Practical Application. Baltimore, Williams & Wilkins, 1995.

Scott, R: Legal and Ethical Issues in Physical Therapy. Gaithersburg, MD, Aspen, 1997.

Self-Assessment

After reviewing the content outlines, the review test items, and the reference list, I have identified my *strengths* in this area to be:

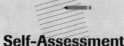

Self-Assessment

After reviewing the content outlines, the review test items, and the reference list, I have identified the following areas in which I need to improve my level of competence:

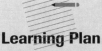

Learning Plan

In order to improve my level of competence, I have identified the following areas of concentrated study, the method(s) by which I will study, and the timelines for each area:

Areas of Concentrated Study:

Learning Plan:

Methods of Study:

Timelines:

Notes

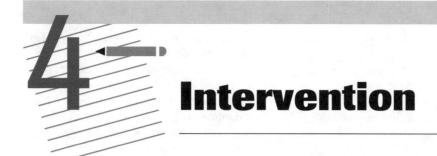

Intervention

In the major content outlines, the Federation of State Boards of Physical Therapy (FSBPT) determined that the Intervention items would constitute 54 percent of the examination. Between 100 and 110 items on the examination are devoted to assessing the ability to safely and effectively implement plans of care for clients evaluated and diagnosed. There are five subsets of competence in the FSBPT content outline under the rubric Intervention: Preparation (10% of the total items), Implementation (23%), Education/Communication/Consultation (7%), Supporting Activities (8%), and System-Specific Procedures (6%).

While reviewing this chapter and the sample test items, a number of questions need to be asked:

- What is the intent?
- What are the expected physiological, biomechanical, and kinesiological changes that should be occurring?
- How is the greatest degree of safety for the client ensured?
- What are the warning signs that necessitate termination or modification of treatment?
- What first aid techniques may be required?
- How will the client be able to incorporate recommendations that affect his or her life, home and work environments, and community?
- What are the ethical and legal obligations in educating and using support staff?
- How can success with client and family home programs be fostered?
- How can other health-care personnel be instructed in safe and efficient tech-

niques appropriate to their scope of practice?
- What are the means for consulting with, referring to, or educating other health-care personnel about physical therapy and individual client progress?
- What are the most effective means of communication with referring practitioners, the health-care team, and other physical therapists?
- What is the best way to serve as a resource for the community in health promotion, screening, and disease prevention?
- What will be the nature of documentation?
- What system-specific procedures must be performed?
- What does the current literature say about specific physical therapy interventions?

As in the preceding chapters, note that the competence statements are the primary considerations, with a substantial number of subsets recurring throughout the content outline. Again, this is an indication of the importance of the item or activity and how it transects multiple activities. The following are the subcontent areas identified by FSBPT under the rubric of Intervention.

PREPARATION

Use strategies to minimize injury to patient and therapist during treatment (such as fall, burn, injury, etc.)
- How to take precautions to reduce client injury from falls
- How to determine the assistance the

client requires during functional activities
- How to manually assist client
- How to protect client while practicing transfer
- Knowledge of proper biomechanical po-

sition for prevention of injuries when transferring clients

- Adapting body position, movements, and equipment to prevent and/or reduce injuries to self

Use appropriate transfer techniques and devices when transferring patients

- Appropriate transfer device for the client
- How to protect client while practicing transfer
- How to place transfer board beneath client to help client move
- Knowledge of proper biomechanical position for prevention of injuries when transferring clients
- Adapting body positions, movements, and equipment to prevent and/or reduce injuries to self

Ensure the safety associated with the use of equipment and modalities and with the environment

- How to monitor the physical space to ensure safe operation
- How to provide protection for the eyes when performing treatments
- How to take precautions to reduce client injury from falls
- How to provide adequate protection for superficial heat treatment
- Safe use and inspection of equipment
- Mechanisms, rationale, and techniques to reduce the potential for transmission of infection
- Adapting body position, movements, and equipment to prevent and/or reduce injuries to self
- Critical evaluation of information related to techniques, equipment, and technology related to client care

Establish and/or evaluate exercise and fitness programs

- Disease processes indication, contraindication, and precautions for treatment/procedures
- Scientific and theoretical basis for various treatments
- Fitness/conditioning/endurance exercise program
- Critical evaluation of information related to techniques, equipment, and technology related to patient care

Position, move, and drape patient for effective, comfortable treatment and privacy

- Position of the client to ensure safety, comfort and modesty, and effectiveness of intervention
- How to position client for comfort, pain or edema control, to increase abnormal tone, and to preserve skin integrity, etc.
- Adapting body position, movements, and equipment to prevent and/or reduce injuries to self

Adjust, revise, or discontinue treatment plan when goals are achieved, patient's status changes, or progress is no longer being demonstrated

- Recognition of signs of physiological distress
- How to integrate findings of multiple test to clarify the client's problem and functional status
- Comparison of client response with target response to determine goal achievement
- How to alter activities in response to client response
- Determination if client's signs/symptoms are indicative of local and/or systemic origin
- Health-care delivery system

Evaluate and recommend changes in work environments for safety and ergonomic design

- Selection of appropriate evaluation tools
- Identification of normal and abnormal posture
- Psychosocial stressors that may affect client response to pain
- Purpose, structure, content, and demonstration of use of various functional tests
- How to question client appropriately to assess cognitive status relative to safety, judgment, and reasoning
- Application of supports at correct sites to achieve goal
- Prescription, fabrication, and use of adaptive equipment
- Appropriate professional verbal and written communication skills
- Resources that may assist clients and families
- Critical evaluation of information related to techniques, equipment, and technology related to client care

Evaluate home, community, and public building environments and recommend modifications for safety and accessibility

- Selection of appropriate evaluation tools
- How to question client appropriately to

assess cognitive status relative to safety, judgment, and reasoning
- How to monitor the physical space to ensure safe operation
- How to take precautions to reduce client injury from falls
- Safe use and inspection of equipment

IMPLEMENTATION

Utilize universal precautions
- Mechanisms, rationale, and techniques to reduce the potential for transmission of infection

Recognize and respond to changes in physiological status (vital signs)
- Signs of life-threatening states (e.g., pulmonary embolus, autonomic dysreflexia)
- Mechanisms, rationale, and techniques to reduce the potential for transmission of infection

Recognize and take measure to remedy blood-sugar level
- Recognition of signs of physiological distress
- First aid and emergency procedures (e.g., stop bleeding, stabilize a fracture, remove foreign particles from skin or eyes)

Administer cardiopulmonary resuscitation
- Signs of life-threatening states (i.e., pulmonary embolus, autonomic dysreflexia)
- CPR procedures
- Mechanisms, rationale, and techniques to reduce the potential for transmission of infection

Apply first aid
- Recognition of allergic reactions to treatment

Utilize the following:

Resisted exercise with and without equipment
- Resisted exercise with and without equipment
- Resisted equipment
- Application of therapeutic exercise

Passive motion/stretching exercise programs
- Passive motion/stretching exercise program
- Application of therapeutic exercise

Balance training
- Home and independent exercise/mobility/safety training programs

- Appropriate professional verbal and written communication skills
- Resources that may assist clients and families
- Critically evaluate information related to techniques, equipment, and technology related to client care

- Signs of life-threatening states (e.g., pulmonary embolism, autonomic dysreflexia)
- First aid and emergency procedures (e.g., stop bleeding, stabilize a fracture, remove foreign particles from skin or eyes)
- Mechanisms, rationale, and techniques to reduce the potential for transmission of infection

Perform treatments to optimize responses with respect to client's schedule for medication or other factors that could influence performance
- Comparison of client response with target response to determine goal achievement
- How to alter activities in response to client response
- Major classes of drugs used in the treatment of musculoskeletal, neurological, cardiovascular, respiratory, and dermal systems
- Appropriate teaching strategies, theories, and techniques to achieve desired goals
- Appropriate, professional verbal and written communication skills
- Critical evaluation of information related to techniques, equipment, and technol-

- Balance training
- How to take precautions to reduce client injury from falls
- How to determine the assistance the client requires during functional activities
- Use of devices such as bolsters, balls, and cylinders
- Application of therapeutic exercise

Fitness/conditioning/endurance exercise programs
- Fitness/conditioning/endurance exercise programs

- Application of therapeutic exercise

Continuous passive motion (CPM)
- Continuous passive motion (CPM)
- Safe use and inspection of equipment
- Application of therapeutic exercise
- How to position client safely on exercise equipment (e.g., treadmill, stationary bicycle)

Home and independent programs
- Home and independent exercise/mobility/safety training programs
- Application of therapeutic exercise

Active and active-assisted exercise
- Active-assisted exercise
- Application of therapeutic exercise

Aquatic exercise/therapeutic pool
- Aquatic exercise/therapeutic pool
- WSI (water safety instructor) certification

Posture training
- Home and independent exercise/mobility/safety training programs
- Posture training
- Use of devices such as bolsters, balls, and cylinders

Relaxation training
- Relaxation training
- How to place a client in position for relaxation exercise
- Identification of appropriate sites for electrode placement

Employ the following to enhance mobility and daily living activities:

Transfers with or without equipment
- Appropriate transfer device for the client
- How to protect client while practicing transfer
- How to place transfer board beneath client to help client move
- Knowledge of proper biomechanical position for prevention of injuries when transferring clients
- Adapting body position, movements, and equipment to prevent and/or reduce injuries to self

Gait training with or without assistive devices
- Underlying impairments that contribute to gait deviations
- Balance training
- How to take precautions to reduce client injury from falls
- How to determine the assistance the client requires during functional activities
- How to place hands/stimulus in position to facilitate or inhibit desired movement
- Measurement and alignment of assistive devices
- Adapting body positions, movements, and equipment to prevent and/or reduce injuries to self

Wheelchair management
- Positional changes or changes in ambulation and wheelchair mobility
- How to determine the assistance the client requires during functional activities

- How to place hands/stimulus in position to facilitate or inhibit desired movement
- Appropriate transfer device for the client
- Measurement and alignment of assistive devices

Bed mobility
- Home and independent exercise/mobility/safety training programs
- How to determine the assistance the client requires during functional activities
- How to manually assist client
- How to place hands/stimulus in position to facilitate or inhibit desired movement
- Application of therapeutic exercise
- Adapting body positions, movement, prostheses, or adaptive devices to client

Adaptive devices, such as orthotics
- Prescription, fabrication, and use of adaptive equipment
- Fabrication of orthotic devices
- Application of orthotics, prostheses, or adaptive devices to client

Work simulation and retraining
- Substitution patterns and synergy patterns
- How to determine the assistance the client requires during functional activities

Personal care activities
- Home and independent exercise/mobility/safety training programs
- How to determine the assistance the client requires during functional activities

Apply the following:

High-voltage stimulation
- High-voltage stimulations
- Effects of modalities used
- Appropriate stimulus and treatment parameters of electrical stimulation
- Electrophysical agents
- Identification of appropriate sites for electrode placement
- Application of electrodes to appropriate site(s)
- Evaluate published studies related to PT practice

Interferential current
- Interferential current
- Effects of modalities used
- Appropriate stimulus and treatment parameters of electrical stimulation
- Electrophysical agents
- Identification of appropriate sites for electrode placement
- Application of electrodes to appropriate site
- Evaluate published studies related to PT practice

Functional electrical nerve stimulation (FES)
- Functional electrical stimulation (FES)
- Effects of modalities used
- Appropriate stimulus and treatment parameters of electrical stimulation
- Electrophysical agents

- Identification of appropriate sites for electrode placement
- Application of electrodes to appropriate site

Low-voltage stimulation
- Low-voltage stimulation
- Effects of modalities used
- Appropriate stimulus and treatment parameters or electrical stimulation
- Electrophysical agents
- Identification of appropriate sites for electrode placement
- Application of electrodes to appropriate site
- Evaluate published studies related to PT practice

Transcutaneous electrical nerve stimulation (TENS)
- Transcutaneous electrical nerve stimulation (TENS)
- Effects of modalities used
- Appropriate stimulus and treatment parameters of electrical stimulation
- Electrophysical agents
- Identification of appropriate sites for electrode placement
- Application of electrodes to appropriate site
- Evaluate published studies related to PT practice

Utilize the following:

Mechanical traction
- Mechanical traction
- Effects of modalities used
- Appropriate mode for mechanical or manual traction
- How to attach belts, straps, and harnesses to client's trunk, pelvis, head, or neck for traction
- Critical evaluation of information related to techniques, equipment, and technology related to patient care

Ultrasound
- Ultrasound
- Critical evaluation of information related to techniques, equipment, and technology related to patient care

Hot pack
- Hot pack
- Effects of modalities used
- How to provide adequate protection for superficial heat treatment

- Critical evaluation of information related to techniques, equipment, and technology related to patient care

Whirlpool/Hubbard tank
- Whirlpool/Hubbard tank
- Operation of whirlpools and surgilavs for wound healing
- Adjustment of aeration and turbulence of hydrotherapy turbine ejectors appropriately for the client's problem
- Mechanisms, rationale, and techniques to reduce the potential for transmission of infection
- Critical evaluation of information related to techniques, equipment, and technology related to client's problem

Cryotherapy/cold packs/ice massage
- Cryotherapy/cold packs/ice massage
- Effects of modalities used
- Critical evaluation of information related

to techniques, equipment, and technology related to client care

Iontophoresis
- Iontophoresis
- Effects of modalities used
- Actions and dosages of medications used in phonophoresis and iontophoresis
- Identification of appropriate sites for electrode placement
- Critical evaluation of information related to techniques, equipment, and technology related to client care

Phonophoresis
- Phonophoresis
- Effects of modalities used
- Actions and dosages of medications used in phonophoresis and iontophoresis
- Identification of appropriate sites for electrode placement
- Critical evaluation of information related to techniques, equipment, and technology related to client care

Mechanical compression/vasopneumatic devices/compression garments
- Mechanical compression/vasopneumatic devices/compression garments
- Effects of modalities used
- Appropriate compression garment
- Critical evaluation of information related to techniques, equipment, and technology related to client care

Paraffin bath
- Paraffin bath
- Effects of modalities used
- How to provide adequate protection for superficial heat treatment
- Critical evaluation of information related to techniques, equipment, and technology related to client care

Short-wave diathermy
- Short-wave diathermy
- Selection of appropriate short-wave applicator
- Identification of appropriate sites for electrode placement
- Critical evaluation of information related to techniques, equipment, and technology related to client care

Ultraviolet light
- Ultraviolet light
- Effects of modalities used
- How to provide protection for the eyes when performing treatment
- Operation and adjustment of electrotherapeutic equipment such as ultraviolet lamps

- Critical evaluation of information related to techniques, equipment, and technology related to client care

Infrared radiation
- Infrared
- Effects of modalities used
- Critical evaluation of information related to techniques, equipment, and technology related to client care

Contrast bath
- Contrast bath
- Critical evaluation of information related to techniques, equipment, and technology related to client care

Biofeedback
- Biofeedback
- Control threshold, gain (sensitivity), and mode of biofeedback
- Identification of appropriate sites for electrode placement
- Critical evaluation of information related to techniques, equipment, and technology related to patient care

Apply flexible dressing/supports/elastic bandaging (e.g., for edema control)
- Application of medication, dressing, bandages, or splints to client's wounds or injuries and for prevention of injuries
- Application of residual limb bandage
- Application of supports at correct sites to achieve goal
- Appropriate compression garment

Guide the patient in normal movement patterns
- Substitution patterns and synergy patterns
- Abnormal reflex patterns
- Concepts of human growth and development from conception to senescence, including physical, cognitive, social, and emotional development
- Direction and grade of movement for the client's movement problem
- How to manually assist client
- How to place hands/stimulus in position to facilitate or inhibit desired movement
- Adapting body position, movements, and equipment to prevent and/or reduce injuries to self

Perform facilitation/inhibition techniques
- How to place hands/stimulus in position to facilitate or inhibit desired movement
- Appropriate joint force
- Application of therapeutic exercise
- How to position client to elicit primitive

reflexes such as Babinski, cremaster, abdominal reflexes

Fabricate and adjust positioning devices
- Application of supports at correct sites to achieve goal
- Measurement and adjustment of assistive devices
- Prescription, fabrication, and use of adaptive equipment
- Fabrication of orthotic devices

Utilize age-appropriate activities to further development
- Concepts of human growth and development from conception to senescence, including physical, cognitive, social, and emotional development

Utilize behavior modification
- Normal and abnormal psychology
- Comparison of client response with target response to determine goal achievement

Apply therapeutic massage
- Identification of different types of massage strokes and their purpose
- Application of hand/fingers with desired pressure, type of movement and direction for chosen massage technique
- Adapting body positions, movements, and equipment to prevent and/or reduce injuries to self

Utilize reality orientation
- Normal and abnormal psychology

Employ the following to enhance mobility and daily living activities:

Energy conservation
- How to alter activities in response to client response
- Home and independent exercise/mobility/safety training programs

- Relaxation training
- How to determine the assistance the client requires during functional activities

EDUCATION/COMMUNICATION/CONSULTATION

Educate support staff in safe and effective handling of patients and equipment related to staff duties
- Appropriate teaching strategies, theories, and techniques to achieve desired goals
- Appropriate, professional verbal and written communication skills
- Adapting body position, movements, and equipment to prevent and/or reduce injuries to self

Educate the client, family/significant others, and other health-care personnel in safe and efficient physical therapy techniques as appropriate
- Appropriate teaching strategies, theories, and techniques to achieve desired goals
- Appropriate, professional verbal and written communication skills
- Adapting body position, movements, and equipment to prevent and/or reduce injuries to self

Educate the client, family/significant others, and other health-care personnel about the post-discharge programs, self-management, and coping strategies
- How to provide clear written instructions with pictures for home programs

- Appropriate teaching strategies, theories, and techniques to achieve desired goals
- Appropriate, professional verbal and written communication skills
- Resources that may assist clients and families
- Health-care delivery system

Instruct the patient clearly and concisely, including the effective use of demonstration
- How to inform clients regarding the purpose and methods of a procedure, what to expect, and what is expected from them
- How to question client appropriately to assess cognitive status relative to safety, judgement, and reasoning
- How to provide clear written instructions with pictures for home programs
- Appropriate teaching strategies, theories, and techniques to achieve desired goals
- Appropriate, professional verbal and written communication skills

Explain physical therapy assessment, treatment procedures, expected outcomes and results to the patient and/or family/significant others and verify their understanding of same
- How to inform clients regarding the purpose and methods of a procedure, what

to expect, and what is expected from them
- Appropriate teaching strategies, theories, and techniques to achieve desired goals
- Appropriate, professional verbal and written communication skills
- Evaluate published studies related to PT practice

Consult with, refer to, or educate other health-care personnel in areas of physical therapy expertise
- Appropriate teaching strategies, theories, and techniques to achieve desired goals
- Appropriate, professional verbal and written communication skills
- Health-care delivery systems

Communicate results of assessment/evaluation to physicians, the health-care team, and other physical therapists
- Objective documentation of treatment, client's status, and progress toward goals
- Appropriate, professional verbal and written communication skills
- Resources that may assist client and families
- Health-care delivery systems

Identify client/family education needs
- How to seek information related to chief complaint, behavior of source of the complaint, aggravating and relieving factors, history of the complaint, medical history, social history during interview
- Appropriate teaching strategies, theories, and techniques to achieve desired goals

SUPPORTING ACTIVITIES

Respect the knowledge, rights, confidentiality, and dignity of the client, family, and significant others
- Models of ethical decision making and bioethics
- Standards of physical therapy practice
- Health-care delivery systems

Abide by regulatory requirements and the legal and ethical standards of the profession
- Models of ethical decision making and bioethics
- Standards of physical therapy practice
- Health-care delivery systems

Recognize the scope and limitations of self and profession
- Standards of physical therapy practice
- Determination whether client's

- Appropriate, professional verbal and written communication skills
- Resources that may assist clients and families

Provide appropriate and timely feedback to patients, families, and colleagues
- Appropriate teaching strategies, theories, and techniques to achieve desired goals
- Appropriate, professional verbal and written communication skills
- Resources that may assist clients and families

Act as a resource to general public regarding health promotion, screening, and disease prevention
- Appropriate, professional verbal and written communication skills
- Mechanisms, rationale, and techniques to reduce the potential for transmission of infection
- Resources that may assist clients and families
- Health-care delivery systems

Document all relevant aspects of care including treatment plan, patient evaluation, and progress notes
- Objective documentation of treatment, client's status, and progress toward goals
- Appropriate, professional verbal and written communication skills
- How to record client data in typical measurement units
- Health-care delivery systems

signs/symptoms are indicative of local and/or systemic origin
- Health-care delivery systems
- Evaluation published studies related to PT practice

Apply principles of ethical decision making
- Models of ethical decision making and bioethics
- Health-care delivery systems

Secure informed consent for evaluation and treatment
- Composition of an informed consent form
- Health-care delivery systems

Procure safe and effective equipment
- Safe use and inspection of equipment
- Principles and practices of management
- Adapting body positions, movements,

and equipment to prevent and/or reduce injuries to self
- Resources that may assist clients and families

Delegate and supervise treatment activities as appropriate

- Education and expected scope of knowledge and responsibility of physical therapist assistants
- Appropriate tasks to be delegated to supportive personnel
- Health-care delivery systems

SYSTEM-SPECIFIC PROCEDURES

Administer oxygen
- How to attach a nasal cannula/O$_2$ mask

- Regulation of the flow of O$_2$ through cannula

Apply the following manual therapy techniques:

Joint mobilization
- Direction and grade of movement for the client's movement problem
- Identification of the contraindications for manual therapy
- Adapting body positions, movements, and equipment to prevent and/or reduce injuries to self

Soft tissue mobilization
- Identification of different types of massage strokes and their purpose
- Application of appropriate techniques for type of soft tissue restriction (e.g.,

fascial release, petrissage, trigger point pressure)
- Adapting body positions, movements, and equipment to prevent and/or reduce injuries to self

Muscle energy
- Factors that effect muscle performance
- Identification of contraindications for manual therapy
- How to place hands/stimulus in position to facilitate or inhibit desired movement
- Adapting body positions, movements, and equipment to prevent and/or reduce injuries to self

Engage in the following prosthetic (amputee) rehabilitation activities:

Residual limb bandaging
- Application of residual limb bandage
- Appropriate compression garment

Preprosthetic training
- Passive motion/stretching exercise program
- Active-assisted exercise
- Fitness/conditioning/endurance exercise programs
- Resisted exercise with and without equipment
- Home and independent exercise/mobility/safety training programs
- Balance training
- Posture training
- Transcutaneous electrical nerve stimulation (TENS)
- Physiology of pressure gradients
- Application of medication, dressing,

bandages, or splints to client's wounds or injuries and for prevention of injuries
- Surgical procedures [knowledge of]
- Identification of tissues to be debrided (granulation vs. necrotic)
- Removal of necrotic tissue with scalpel, scissors, tweezers, gauze

Prosthetic gait training
- Application of orthotics, prostheses, or adaptive devices to client
- How to place client's residual limb in socks, sleeve, and prosthesis

Care and use of prosthesis
- Application of orthotics, prostheses, or adaptive devices to client
- How to place client's residual limb in socks, sleeve, and prosthesis
- How to provide clear written instructions with pictures for home programs

Utilize the following for pulmonary secretion removal:

Instillation/suctioning
- Human anatomy and physiology
- How to place a suction catheter for endotracheal suctioning
- How to obtain culture specimens by probing tissue with swag, inserting suction catheter into trachea
- Mechanisms, rationale, and techniques to reduce the potential for transmission of infection

Bronchial drainage techniques
- Application of vibratory force with hands over client's thorax in coordination with breathing
- How to position hands to perform percussion, vibration, and shaking techniques
- Application of cupped hand to client's thorax for bronchial drainage

- Mechanisms, rationale, and techniques to reduce the potential for transmission of infection
- Adapting body positions, movements, and equipment to prevent and/or reduce injuries to self

Cough enhancement techniques
- Application of vibratory force with hands over client's thorax in coordination with breathing
- Application of pressure to extrathoracic trachea, mid-abdomen, lower costal border, or proximal sites to enhance cough
- Mechanisms, rationale, and techniques to reduce the potential for transmission of infection

Mechanical devices to loosen secretions
- Safe use of equipment

Utilize the following to enhance respiration:

Positions to relieve dyspnea
- Positioning of the client to ensure safety, comfort and modesty, and effectiveness of intervention
- Relaxation training

Positions to improve ventilation/oxygenation
- Positioning of client to ensure safety, comfort and modesty, and effectiveness of intervention

Breathing exercise
- How to place hands/stimulus in position to facilitate or inhibit desired movement

- Application of vibratory force with hands over client's thorax in coordination with breathing
- How to place hands on epigastric and upper chest area to demonstrate air shifts by cueing

Respiratory muscle training with functional activities
- How to determine the assistance the client requires during functional activities
- How to place hands/stimulus in position to facilitate or inhibit desired movement

Incentive spirometry

Perform wound cleansing and debride wounds
- Identification of tissues to be debrided (granulation vs. necrotic)
- Removal of necrotic tissue with scalpel, scissors, tweezers, gauze
- Mechanisms, rationale, and techniques to reduce the potential for transmission of infection
- Adapting body positions, movements, and equipment to prevent and/or reduce injuries to self

Apply wound coverings
- Wound status and signs of inflammation and/or healing
- Application of medication, dressing,

bandages, or splints to client's wounds or injuries and for protection of self
- First aid and emergency procedures (e.g., stop bleeding, stabilize a fracture, remove foreign particles from skin or eyes)
- Mechanisms, rationale, and techniques to reduce the potential for transmission of infection

Apply scar management techniques
- Phases of connective tissue repair and scar tissue formation
- Appropriate scar management technique (e.g., friction massage pressure garments, gel pads)

- Appropriate pressure garment

Provide vestibular rehabilitation
- Appropriate vestibular techniques

Provide oral-motor stimulation
- How to place hands/stimulus in position to facilitate or inhibit desired movement

Fabricate and adjust orthoses
- Fabrication of orthotic devices

- Application of orthotics, prostheses, or adaptive devices to client

Utilize taping techniques
- Application of medication, dressing, bandages, or splints to client's wounds or injuries and for prevention of injuries
- Application of supports at correct sites to achieve goal

INTENT OF CONTENT SECTION

For the physical therapist and the client, intervention for the management of movement dysfunctions is the major content area. The relative weight of 54% of the items speaks to the importance and valuing of the various interventions physical therapists are legally permitted to provide. These items represent a synthesis of

- anatomy
- physiology
- neuroanatomy
- neurophysiology
- life span

- clinical decision-making processes, and
- the selection and administration, either directly or through delegation, of techniques, procedures, and modalities for the alleviation of symptoms.

It involves knowledge and skill insofar as any written examination can. The licensure examination seeks to obtain evidence that the individual physical therapist *is* competent and will safely and effectively provide care that is directed at prevention, alleviation, and correction of movement dysfunctions to the degree possible considering both the medical and pathokinesiological diagnoses.

The intent of this content area is to ensure that services are provided in a manner that is ethical, legal, and cost-effective. The items that reflect this content area require demonstration of knowledge, comprehension, and the ability to apply, synthesize, analyze, and evaluate information. In addition to the initial three sample questions, there are 200 items included in this chapter. Examples of test items in this content area include:

EXAMPLE #1:
When performing PAs to the cervical spine unilaterally, it is essential that the line of force being applied is:

A. perpendicular to the horizontal plane
B. angled medially
C. equal over each vertebra
D. sufficient to elicit p1

The correct response is A. The correct vertebral movement can only be obtained by applying pressure in a straight line.

EXAMPLE #2:
During a treatment session with a client in an outpatient setting, the client complains of crushing chest pain and collapses. Vital signs are monitored, and there is no heart beat. The most appropriate action to take is to:

A. first telephone the paramedics
B. initiate cardiopulmonary resuscitation (CPR)

C. call for help
D. direct the assistant to telephone the paramedics

The correct response is D. The paramedics should be called quickly and almost simultaneously CPR should be initiated.

EXAMPLE #3:
As a program of care is initiated, it is essential that the client understand what is intended, how the process will be accomplished, and what the potential risks are before the treatment program is begun. This is referred to as:

A. professional courtesy
B. informed consent
C. beneficence
D. nonmaleficence

The correct response is B. This is both an ethical and legal requirement in contemporary practice.

SAMPLE TEST ITEMS COVERING INTERVENTION CONTENT

Please read each item carefully and anticipate the correct response. Then carefully look for the correct response in the choices provided. The correct answers are included at the end of the chapter.

1. **A client is being treated with ultrasonography, which can be effectively applied to an area:**

   A. five times (50% the size) of the effective radiating area (ERA)
   B. equal to the size of the ERA
   C. two times the size of the ERA
   D. three times the size of the ERA

2. **Which one of the following accurately describes the relationship of the thermal effects of ultrasonography?**

   A. increase frequency, decrease heating
   B. decrease protein, increase heating
   C. decrease blood flow, decrease heating
   D. increase reflection, increase heating

3. **When is muscle play not an appropriate choice to treat injured muscle tissue?**

   A. in the acute stage
   B. in the subacute stage
   C. in the chronic stage
   D. when lengthening is desired

4. **If the purpose in applying massage is the reduction of edema:**

   A. always precede the massage with ice packs.
   B. begin proximally and proceed distally to proximally.
   C. use it in conjunction with ultraviolet therapy.
   D. follow the massage with superficial heat.

5. **Which one of the following is a contraindication to stretching?**

   A. decreased ROM because of adhesions
   B. muscle weakness
   C. bony block to joint motion
   D. muscle length imbalance

6. **While treating a chronic strain of the right gluteal muscles of a 79-year-old client with soft tissue mobilization:**

   A. Position the client in right sidelying.
   B. Decrease the treatment duration because the reflex arc is more sensitive and the fullest effect is obtained rapidly.
   C. Treat the right gluteal muscles along with the lumbar paraspinals, hamstrings, and gastrocnemius/soleus muscles on the right side.
   D. Treat the patient primarily with effleurage secondary to the stage and age of the patient.

7. **Autogenic inhibition is:**

   A. a factor that may enhance muscle stretching
   B. a precaution in muscle stretching of aging clients
   C. a method of inhibiting the tight muscle by eliciting a contraction of its antagonist muscle
   D. present in clients with neurologic dysfunctions whose muscles have been overstretched

8. **All of the following are appropriate ways of manipulating exercise parameters during a session to promote endurance using heavy-duty rubber bands except:**

   A. decreasing rest intervals between contractions
   B. increasing the number of repetitions
   C. increasing the duration of contractions
   D. increasing the tensile strength of the rubber band

9. **The most accurate description of the technique *timing for emphasis* is:**

   A. giving a quick stretch at the beginning of the pattern
   B. passively moving the limb through the pattern
   C. holding back all but one of the components of the pattern
   D. resisting patterns in positions other than supine

10. **While using the proprioceptive neuromuscular facilitation (PNF) upper extremity (UE) extension and abduction pattern, the wrist component is:**

    A. extension and radial deviation
    B. extension and ulnar deviation
    C. flexion and radial deviation
    D. flexion and ulnar deviation

11. **Hold-relax, as officially referred to in the PNF literature:**

    A. is synonymous with contract-relax in its description
    B. uses vigorous isometric holds to increase ROM
    C. uses gentle isometric holds to increase ROM
    D. is mostly applied as a pain reduction technique for clients with hemiparesis

12. **For a client who lacks eccentric control of scapular posterior elevation musculature, which of the following PNF patterns would best address the problem?**

    A. resisted UE D2 extension pattern with tubing attached at client's foot
    B. resisted UE D1 flexion pattern with tubing attached at client's foot
    C. resisted UE D2 flexion pattern with tubing attached above client's head
    D. resisted UE D1 extension pattern with tubing attached above client's head

13. **A 36-year-old construction worker who sustained a lumbar injury is participating in a work-hardening program. All of the following are typical components of the program except:**

    A. work simulation
    B. body mechanics education
    C. management of symptoms of pain
    D. functional capacity evaluation and reevaluation

14. **Which one of the following statements is an example of the relaxation technique of *neuromuscular dissociation*?**

    A. "Tense your right biceps while keeping all of the rest of your muscles relaxed."
    B. "See yourself lying on a warm, sunny beach. As each wave rolls out to the sea, you slowly let go of the tension in your forearm."
    C. "As I touch your right biceps, let the tension melt and roll out of your arm."
    D. "Repeat to yourself 'My right arm is heavy. My right arm is warm. My right arm is completely relaxed.' and repeat this process for 3 to 5 minutes."

15. **A 45-year-old client complains of low back pain (LBP) with radiating pain down the back of the left leg to the ankle. Pain has been present for 12 days. On the initial visit, part of the treatment consisted of lumbar static traction in the supine position for 10 minutes. It is now 2 days later, and the client reports that the symptoms are the same. It is decided that traction is still indicated. Which one of the following traction parameters would be appropriate at this time?**

    A. 50 lbs for 5 minutes
    B. 60 lbs for 20 minutes
    C. 90 lbs for 10 minutes
    D. 100 lbs for 15 minutes

16. The client described in item 15 returns for the third visit and states that the symptoms increased after the last visit. Which one of the following traction settings would be appropriate during this visit?

   A. 45 lbs for 10 minutes
   B. 60 lbs for 15 minutes
   C. 80 lbs for 10 minutes
   D. 90 lbs for 15 minutes

17. A 46-year-old public health nurse carried a heavy portable electrocardiography machine on the right shoulder to and from the car and several patients' homes 2 weeks ago. Client reports being awakened that night by severe LBP, right leg pain, and numbness in the right foot. Has not worked for 2 weeks. Pain has decreased in intensity with decreased activity; however, LBP, right lower extremity (RLE) pain, and right foot numbness persist. There is no other history of injury. Bilateral straight-leg raises (SLRs) elicit LBP as the lumbar spine moves. While standing, posture reflects bilateral hip and knee flexion, hip adduction, and genu valgum. Movements are still guarded and tentative. The lumbopelvic region is still tender to bilateral palpation. The client reports a decrease in pain with grade II manual traction but complains of increased pain with grade III. Based on this information, today it is appropriate to apply:

   A. manual traction without tissue stretch
   B. manual traction with tissue stretch short of end range
   C. manual traction with tissue stretch to end of physiological range
   D. mechanical traction to one-half of body weight

18. For the client in item 17, instruction in correct sitting posture should also be included in today's treatment. The client should be advised to **not** engage in:

   A. reclined sitting
   B. erect sitting
   C. slump sitting
   D. forward sitting

19. The client being treated is a 50-year-old secretary who spends at least 50% of the day at a computer. The rest of the workday is spent filing and at the telephone. The condition is diagnosed as a C6 nerve root irritation from the C5–6 disc. During the first treatment session, the client was treated with traction and was pain free for 4 hours after treatment. The symptoms returned, but they were less intense. The traction intervention is being repeated with one parameter changed. Which of the following parameters would be the most logical?

   A. Change the position of the client during traction.
   B. Increase the time.
   C. Increase the weight.
   D. Change the head halter to Saunder's attachment.

20. While using PNF for a client, you should apply manual contact for resisting the anterior elevation pattern of the pelvis. Resistance is limited to the:

   A. iliac crest just above the ASIS
   B. level of the ASIS
   C. ischial tuberosity
   D. trochanter of the femur

21. Which PNF technique should be used to teach a patient a pattern of movement?

   A. traction
   B. rotation
   C. rhythmic initiation
   D. slow reversals

22. When resisting a lengthening contraction of the pelvic anterior elevation pattern in PNF, the verbal command should be:

   A. "Hold it there; don't let me move you."
   B. "Move with me slowly but constantly."
   C. "Sit down and back into my hand."
   D. "Make me work to pull you back."

23. When considering a client's movement during a PNF session, the pelvic pattern during the midswing phase of gait on the swing leg side is most accurately described as:

A. posterior depression
B. anterior elevation
C. posterior elevation
D. anterior depression

24. An elderly client being treated at bedside 1 day after surgical pinning of a left hip fracture has a 25% partial weight-bearing status on the left and has not been out of bed. In preparation for gait, which procedure(s) can be performed to maximize muscle activity and contraction of the LLE without compromising fracture healing while the client is supine in bed?

A. approximation through the left heel and concurrently resisting hip abduction on the right
B. approximation through the left heel and concurrently resisting hip abduction on the left
C. approximation through the left heel and concurrently resisting hip rotation on the left
D. approximation through the right (uninvolved) heel only

25. A client was referred for treatment of LBP secondary to a strain of the iliolumbar ligament. The pain is subacute, but the client continues to move very stiffly because of excessive muscle splinting. Maximum pain level is 5 on a scale of 10. The most appropriate initial technique while working with pelvic patterns would be:

A. slow reversals to improve active movement
B. rhythmic initiation to encourage muscle relaxation
C. combined isotonics to encourage muscle relaxation
D. passive movement only

26. A client is to be instructed in lumbar extension exercises. As part of the planning for this session, it is essential that the physical therapist:

A. be an expert in demonstrating the skill.
B. delineate the steps involved as in a task analysis.
C. explain all of the steps involved in the exercise.
D. gain full mastery of the exercise by the end of today's session.

27. In the middle of a treatment session, a 13-year-old client with a diagnosis of T-12 paraplegia begins to talk about the automobile accident that resulted in the injury. Because the other occupants of the car were killed, little information has been available. For the first time, it is learned that one passenger was a gang member and that the car was deliberately run off the road on a hillside by members of a rival gang. Before this conversation, the client was not able to learn and perform strengthening exercises, transfer training, and activities of daily living (ADLs). According to Maslow's hierarchy of needs, the client may be experiencing difficulty in learning because his _____ needs have not been met.

A. self-actualization
B. love and respect
C. safety and survival
D. self-esteem

28. Appropriate timing in giving feedback to persons learning psychomotor skills is described by motor learning theorists as:

A. constructive input
B. knowledge of results
C. outcome measures
D. integrative processing

29. **When teaching a client who has undergone a total hip replacement to perform a functional activity, such as transferring from sitting to standing, what domain will be the primary goal or objective (according to Bloom)?**

    A. cognitive
    B. integrative
    C. affective
    D. psychomotor

30. **A 70-year-old client with a fractured hip underwent internal fixation. Today's treatment goal is to instruct the caregiver in assisted transfers in preparation for discharge to home. In order to increase the probability that both of them will perform the transfers correctly, the home instruction should include:**

    A. an illustrated handout
    B. an audiotape of your verbal instructions
    C. a videotape of transfer techniques
    D. the department's telephone number in case they have questions

31. **As the supervising therapist for inpatient services in a skilled nursing facility (SNF), it is noticed that one of the therapists is shouting at a client and repeating instructions rapidly. The client appears to be becoming confused and less able to perform the exercise program. The therapist is told that the client must have time to practice without continuous feedback and that the tone of voice needs to be calmer and quieter. The rationale for these instructions is:**

    A. There is a difference between performance and learning.
    B. Timing of feedback is critical for learning to occur.
    C. The client is emotionally upset with the therapy session.
    D. The therapist seems to be acting condescendingly toward the client.

32. **A client asks what level of education the physical therapist assistant had before joining the staff. The correct response is:**

    A. an associate's degree from an accredited program
    B. a baccalaureate degree from an accredited program
    C. a certificate of completion from an accredited institution
    D. a high school diploma and completion of a vocational technical program

33. **The client in item 32 then asks if the treating physical therapist has a license as a physical therapist. The response is that the therapist recently graduated from a master of physical therapy degree program and took the examination 2 weeks ago. By law, the therapist is considered to be a:**

    A. registered physical therapist
    B. nonregistered physical therapist
    C. physical therapist license applicant
    D. licensed physical therapist

34. **The client in items 32 and 33 asks how someone knows whether an education program for physical therapists is of acceptable quality. The most appropriate reply is that education programs are subject to:**

    A. certification
    B. state approval
    C. regional accreditation
    D. specialized accreditation

35. **In some states, physical therapists are permitted to evaluate and treat clients without a referral from a physician. This is commonly referred to as:**

    A. autonomy
    B. direct access
    C. independent practice
    D. professional status

36. The ability to recognize and to some extent share the emotions and states of mind of another is:

A. association
B. empathy
C. sympathy
D. understanding

37. The method of payment for the services for a client currently receiving treatment has an established maximum dollar amount for services provided. This method of payment is commonly referred to as:

A. capitation
B. rationing
C. fee for service
D. indemnification

38. Prepaid group practices have dramatically increased in numbers in the past decade. These practices are known as:

A. preferred provider organizations
B. prospective payment systems
C. health maintenance organizations
D. community-based insurance companies

39. When a provider of care is forced to make a decision that violates one of the principles of ethics in order to adhere to another of the principles, the situation is referred to as:

A. a moral conflict
B. an ethical issue
C. maleficence
D. an ethical dilemma

40. A physical therapist has been observed documenting treatments that were not given. Your obligation as a licensed physical therapist is to:

A. confront the behavior and report to the facility administrator.
B. report the therapist to the licensing agency.
C. request termination of employment of the offending therapist.
D. report the overcharges to the client's payors.

41. The clinic has too many clients for the available staff resources, and a priority system is needed to distribute services among the potential clients. This involves:

A. beneficence
B. fidelity
C. veracity
D. justice

42. When applying electrical stimulation, attention is paid to motor points. These are sites:

A. on the skin surface where the underlying muscle can be electrically stimulated
B. directly over the underlying muscle belly
C. that correspond to the acupuncture points for needle insertion
D. for placement of surface electrodes for electroneuromyographic testing

43. When a muscle contracts in response to stimulation with galvanic (direct) current but not in response to faradic (alternating) current, the phenomenon is referred to as:

A. denervation
B. rheobase response
C. reaction to degeneration
D. regeneration

44. In applying conventional transcutaneous electrical nerve stimulation (TENS), the pulse duration (width) and the frequency (rate) settings are:

A. 150–250 μsec and 1–4 Hz
B. 20–60 μsec and 50–500 Hz
C. 100–200 μsec and 2–3 Hz
D. 150–250 μsec and 100 Hz

45. When interferential current is applied, the waveform is:

A. twin peak pulses
B. continuous sine wave
C. direct
D. sine wave

46. In administering low-voltage electrical stimulation, the intensity is:

A. less than 150 volts
B. 90–100 mA
C. 150–175 volts
D. 70–90 mA

47. Brunnstrom's treatment theory is used in providing therapeutic exercise for a client who suffered a cerebrovascular accident (CVA). Accordingly, when the client demonstrates synergy patterns:

A. Encourage the client to stay out of the synergy pattern.
B. This pattern has minimal relevance to the exercise.
C. The client should bear weight through the extremity to normalize tone.
D. Use the strong components of the synergy to facilitate activation of weaker muscles for function.

48. A client is just beginning to demonstrate return of movement within a flexor synergy pattern in her UE. Brunnstrom techniques are being used. Which of the following should be used?

A. scapular techniques to facilitate elevation and retraction because these are often the first motions to return within the synergy pattern
B. rowing in and out of flexor synergy, emphasizing the movement out of synergy in order to facilitate normal movement patterns
C. finger extension techniques (rolling, swatting, molding) to facilitate finger extension because normal movement patterns return in distal areas before proximal areas
D. any of the above three techniques are appropriate for this client at this stage of recovery

49. In working with a client who experienced a CVA, a Marie-Foix response is elicited. This occurred as a result of:

A. dorsiflexion, eversion, plantarflexion
B. plantarflexion, inversion, dorsiflexion
C. inversion, plantarflexion, knee flexion
D. plantarflexion, eversion, dorsiflexion

50. A progression of PNF techniques based on developmental strategies to improve motor control would be:

A. rhythmic stabilization, slow reversals, rhythmic initiation, repeated contraction
B. prone on elbows, one-leg stance, quadruped, kneeling
C. rhythmic initiation, rhythmic stabilization, slow reversals
D. sidelying supine, long sitting, prone, quadruped

51. Which of the following is not true about managing secondary complications of spinal cord injury (SCI)?

A. Examine the skin for redness and do periodic pressure relief techniques.
B. During autonomic dysreflexia, remove restrictive clothing and have the client lie down.
C. Use stretching to combat heterotopic bone formation.
D. Use abdominal binders and long support stockings to prevent orthostatic hypotension.

52. The client is a 25-year-old with a medical diagnosis of multiple sclerosis (MS). The progression of exercises has been developed. The caregivers are being instructed in carrying out a home program that would include the following in a half-lying position:

1) lower extremity (LE) (hip) abduction with knee flexed
2) heel of LE to opposite LE toe, ankle, shin, and knee
3) unilateral LE flexion and extension with foot off mat or floor
4) bilateral reciprocal LE flexion and extension

What is the correct progression of the four exercises?

A. 1, 3, 4, 2
B. 3, 4, 2, 1
C. 1, 3, 2, 4
D. 3, 1, 2, 4

53. **Yesterday an 82-year-old who suffered a CVA was evaluated. The three main problems to be addressed include decreased balance, decreased active range of motion (AROM) in the left lower leg (LLL), and dependence in all functional activities. The appropriate choice of techniques and position for strengthening trunk extensors is:**

A. Brunnstrom: forward flexion with arms cradled, semi-sitting
B. PNF: approximation through the shoulders, adding RS in sitting
C. rowing in synergy with resistance only in the extension direction
D. NDT: align and then facilitate standing weight shift in diagonals

54. **For the client in item 53, it is now 2 weeks later, and trunk extension work continues. The most appropriate of the following techniques and positions would be:**

A. Brunnstrom: assisted forward flexion with arms cradled, sitting
B. PNF: chopping pattern in supine
C. Swiss ball sitting activities
D. both A and C because they would facilitate greater gain

55. **A 52-year-old client with hemiplegia is being gait trained. What is the most appropriate sequence of activities to be used to progress from easier to harder tasks?**

A. lateral weight shift; single leg stance; diagonal weight shift; side stepping
B. lateral weight shift; diagonal weight shift; single leg stance; braiding
C. stride weight shifts; lateral weight shifts; side stepping; single leg stance
D. lateral weight shifts; single leg stance; side stepping; hip hiking

56. **A client in the intensive care unit (ICU) is 21 years old, has suffered a head injury, and now has a chest tube in place. It has been decided that sensory stimulation is appropriate. All of the following are true except:**

A. An appropriate auditory stimulation would be to leave the radio or TV on for background sounds.
B. Motor responses, such as eye movements, facial grimacing, changes in posture, head turning, or vocalization, should be recorded.
C. Sensory stimulation is theorized to activate the reticular activating system, causing a general increase in arousal.
D. Vestibular stimulation can be provided by neck ROM exercises, rolling on the bed, rocking, or pushing the client in a wheelchair.

57. **Treatment considerations for agitated head-injured patients include:**

A. use of simple, one-step commands and speaking in short, simple sentences
B. touching the patients often to calm them
C. keeping sessions short and allowing for frequent rest periods
D. A and C should be included

58. **According to the Rancho Los Amigos stage of cognitive function, if the client appears oriented to place but performs ADLs in a robot-like way and requires at least minimal supervision for safety, the cognitive level is:**

A. stage III, localized response
B. stage VII, automatic and appropriate
C. stage VIII, unsafe, appropriate
D. stage IV, purposeful, oriented

59. **In treating a 34-year-old client who demonstrates hemiplegia secondary to a CHI while rock climbing, it is noted that all of the following are true about the client's condition except:**

    A. The flaccidity that follows the acute episode is sooner or later replaced by spasticity.
    B. Each of the four limb synergies incorporates specific movement components regardless of whether the synergy is elicited reflexively or performed voluntarily.
    C. The flexor synergy is typically the weaker of the two lower extremity synergies and is dominated by hip flexion.
    D. Associated movements cannot be elicited in a limb that is essentially flaccid.

60. **Three of four clients demonstrated visual or perceptual disturbance. This was consistent with the literature, which indicates that these disturbances are common in individuals with these diagnoses. Patients with _____ do not experience visual or perceptual disturbances.**

    A. SCI
    B. CVA
    C. TIA
    D. MS

61. **The client has a medical diagnosis of osteoarthritis and has been instructed in a home exercise program to maintain ROM and strength. Paraffin bath has been included in the treatment plan. The primary purpose for this is to:**

    A. facilitate movement
    B. decrease inflammation
    C. alleviate pain
    D. promote ROM

62. **A 2-year-old client has had a sacro-coccygeal teratoma surgically removed. The child's mother asks what her daughter's prognosis is. The ethical and legal response is:**

    A. "I can't answer that for you. Only the physician can discuss this with you."
    B. "Have you spoken with your physician about her future? Most of these tumors are benign."
    C. "I don't really know and can't answer your question."
    D. "There are several books in the medical library that you might want to check out so you will know for yourself."

63. **A 12-year-old girl with a medical diagnosis of cystic fibrosis (CF) is a client. The medical center is involved in a *CFTR* gene therapy project. This may result in a different approach on the part of physical therapists in the management of clients with CF. This is because the *CFTR* gene:**

    A. corrects the chloride defect in cells
    B. eliminates the risk of infections in clients with CF
    C. ensures a life expectancy of 40 years
    D. reverses all previous damage caused by CF

64. **A physical therapy aide has been accepted into a physical therapy education program and asks for your experiences in assessing ROMs and muscle strength. The ethical and legal response is to:**

    A. ask one of the therapists or assistants to become the aide's mentor.
    B. agree to provide such learning experiences under supervision.
    C. refer the assistant to another therapist who has supervised aides in the past.
    D. deny the request because it would be a violation of the law.

65. As a member of the primary care team for clients with an SCI, a discussion is in process regarding weaning a client from a ventilator. Which ventilator mode would immediately precede progression to continuous positive airway pressure (CPAP)?

A. synchronized intermittent mandatory ventilation (SIMV)
B. assist control
C. control
D. assist

66. The client being seen this afternoon has severe rotatory scoliosis. The flow volume pattern on pulmonary function testing can be expected to be:

A. normal
B. restrictive
C. related to chronic obstructive pulmonary disease (COPD)
D. similar to emphysema

67. Which of the following is **not** a contraindication to percussion during postural drainage?

A. rib fracture
B. hemothorax
C. sonorous rhonchi
D. empyema

68. A client with COPD uses sternocleidomastoids during quiet inspiration. Which of the following would be the best treatment with which to start today?

A. Use postural drainage with percussion.
B. Encourage the patient to cough.
C. Teach diaphragmatic breathing.
D. Teach pursed-lip breathing.

69. A client is lying in bed. Respiratory rate is 40, left ankle and leg edema are present, and there are positive results for Homan's sign. His body temperature is 98.6°F. What is the most likely cause of the tachypnea given the following choices?

A. cor pulmonale
B. pneumonia
C. emphysema
D. pulmonary embolus

70. The client has a pulmonary-related movement dysfunction. In preparation for the treatment session today, sonorous rhonchi in both lungs were auscultated. Which of the following interventions is indicated?

A. Use postural drainage with percussion.
B. Encourage the client to cough.
C. Teach diaphragmatic breathing.
D. Teach pursed-lip breathing.

71. The client has a diagnosis of COPD, has been hospitalized for 3 days, and is now ready for discharge. Physical therapy is requested for a pre-discharge assessment. The interview reveals that the client lives alone. The client ambulated short distances independently before admission and has no stairs into or in the house. Client's SaO_2 level at rest on 2 L of oxygen by nasal cannula is 97%. During treatment, the client ambulates slowly on room air for 50 feet independently and is mildly short of breath and fatigued after walking. SaO_2 level on room air after ambulation is 92%. Which of the following would be the best discharge plan?

A. The client should be discharged home with supplemental oxygen and instructions on energy conservation techniques.
B. The client should be discharged home without supplemental oxygen and with instructions on energy conservation techniques.
C. The client should have SNF for physical therapy with supplemental oxygen and instructions on energy conservation techniques.
D. The client should stay in bed with instructions on energy conservation techniques.

72. **Three reflexes have been identified as potentially affecting the diameter of the thoracic outlet and the blood flow to the UE. The most common and most frequently overlooked dysfunctional reflex is:**

    A. a paradoxical breathing pattern
    B. the flexion-withdrawal reflex
    C. vasoconstriction
    D. vasodilatation

73. **When using the McConnell taping system in the treatment of a client with patellofemoral syndrome:**

    A. the tape should be applied with the knee in about 40 degrees of flexion
    B. the abnormal tilt component should be corrected before the glide
    C. the abnormal rotation component is corrected last
    D. B and C

74. **After evaluation, it is determined that the client has an anteriorly rotated right ilium that contributes to symptoms of pain. Which of the following would be appropriate in a home program?**

    A. isometric contractions of the right hip flexors and left hip extensors
    B. using the gluteus minimus by positioning the left hip in 90 degrees flexion, abducted and externally rotated and resisting in adduction
    C. isometric contractions of the left hip flexors and the right hip extensors
    D. isotonic trunk rotation to the right

75. **The client is a professional athlete. The treatment program is intended to prevent future shoulder separations. Which is the primary structure for prevention of shoulder separations?**

    A. inferior acromioclavicular ligament
    B. trapezoid portion of coracoclavicular ligament
    C. supraspinatus tendon
    D. conoid portion of coracoclavicular ligament

76. **An exercise program is designed to strengthen the musculature for depression of the humerus on the glenoid. The primary muscle involved is the:**

    A. pectoralis major
    B. pectoralis minor
    C. subclavius
    D. supraspinatus

77. **The client has limited UE elevation. The evaluation revealed limited clavicular elevation. The plan of care includes mobilization of the sternoclavicular joint. Which of the following accessory movements would accomplish this task?**

    A. anterior to posterior
    B. posterior to anterior
    C. rostral to caudal
    D. caudal to rostral

78. **As a client approaches the end of a therapeutic exercise session, muscle fatigue is observed. This means that the _____ strain on bone is _____.**

    A. tensile/increased
    B. tensile/decreased
    C. compressive/increased
    D. stress/increased

79. **It is important to reduce unilateral tight hamstrings because it can contribute to a/an:**

    A. ipsilateral lateral tilt of the pelvis
    B. contralateral backward posterosuperior iliac spine (PSIS)
    C. ipsilateral forward ASIS
    D. ipsilateral backward pelvic torsion (tilt)

80. **Stretching exercises for which of the following reduce a lumbar flexion restriction?**

    A. erector spinae and hamstrings
    B. hamstrings and psoas
    C. psoas and erector spinae
    D. psoas and gluteals

81. **Torque is greatest while applying resistance to a client when:**

    A. the moment arm is longest
    B. the action line of the muscles you are using are furthest from your axis of motion
    C. you apply force perpendicular to the lever arm
    D. all of the above

82. **During treatment of a 48-year-old writer with a musculoskeletal dysfunction involving the scapular musculature, a technique is used in which the client is asked to attempt to find the point on the back where the therapist's finger is touching and allow the tightness to melt like butter. This is an example of:**

    A. superficial myofascial release
    B. deep myofascial release
    C. craniosacral alignment
    D. creative visualization

83. **As active assistance range of motion (AAROM) of the left upper extremity (LUE) is performed, clavicular elevation is limited. Which structure is responsible for the limitation?**

    A. coracoclavicular ligament
    B. coracohumeral ligament
    C. costoclavicular ligament
    D. articular disc

84. **In a strengthening exercise program involving manual resistance and forceful adduction of the arm, the pull of the teres major on the scapula is stabilized by which muscles?**

    A. serratus anterior
    B. rhomboids
    C. deltoid
    D. trapezius

85. **An exercise program developed for a client involves maximal knee extension strengthening. What normally limits knee extension?**

    A. soft tissue compression
    B. posterior capsule
    C. patella compressing on femoral condyles
    D. collateral ligaments

86. **A client is working on an exercise program developed to decrease tight hamstrings. Gait before initiation of the program was characterized by:**

    A. shortened stride length
    B. lumbar spine flexion
    C. posterior pelvic tilt
    D. all of the above

87. **In the case of a client who underwent arthroscopic removal of a torn medial meniscus, instruction is given to perform standing quadriceps exercises. During performance of the exercise program, normal biomechanical motion at the knee is observed. The movement at the knee is:**

    A. femur rolls forward and then glides back
    B. femur rolls back then and glides forward
    C. tibia rolls forward and then glides back
    D. tibia rolls back and then glides forward

88. **Which of the following exercises is most specific for strengthening the abdominal muscles?**

    A. bilateral SLRs
    B. straight-legged sit-ups
    C. curl-ups with hips and knees at 90 degrees over chair
    D. hooked lying sit-ups

89. **Intervention is directed at bilaterally lengthening the suboccipital muscles. The client has compensated for this shortening by:**

    A. cervical side bending
    B. flexion at the lower cervical spine
    C. opening the jaw
    D. extending the lumbar spine

90. In developing an exercise program for a client who has restrictions through the neck and back, consideration should be taken that the area with more flexion and extension is the:

    A. mid-cervical spine
    B. mid-thoracic spine
    C. thoracolumbar junction
    D. lumbar spine

91. The client has marked interosseous weakness. Of the following activities included in an exercise program, which will be most affected by the weakness?

    A. cylindrical grip
    B. spherical grip
    C. hook grip
    D. pinch grip

92. A client demonstrated weak upper limb abduction but normal ROM and weak and limited active flexion (0 to 130 degrees) with normal passive range. The exercise program will be targeted to increase the strength of which muscle?

    A. trapezius
    B. deltoid
    C. serratus anterior
    D. pectoralis major

93. A client has an infection in the right lung and bronchi. Which of the following postures will drain the right lobes?

    A. lying on the left side
    B. lying supine
    C. lying on the right side
    D. sitting erect

94. The quadriceps generates maximal isometric tension at _____ _____ degrees of flexion because _____.

    A. 45/this is the point in the range where its moment arm is longest
    B. 60/this is the point in the range where its length-to-tension ratio is greatest
    C. 45/this is the point in the range where its length-to-tension ratio is greatest
    D. 60/this is the point in the range where its moment arm is longest

95. After implementing an exercise program for a client with knee flexion contracture of 20 degrees, the one activity that is still most affected by the contracture is:

    A. tying shoes
    B. going down stairs (involved leg as trail leg)
    C. sitting in a straight-backed chair
    D. stance phase of gait

96. An exercise program has the peroneus longus and tibialis posterior function as a force couple. Which motion will the client be performing?

    A. plantarflexion
    B. inversion
    C. dorsiflexion
    D. eversion

97. While manually performing resisted right hip external rotation and passive right hip internal rotation, a client complains of pain down the right posterior calf and into the heel. The same exercise is performed on the right but with the knee extended; the pain intensifies. Resisted hip extension and resisted knee flexion are both pain free. These findings are suggestive of:

    A. hamstring strain
    B. piriformis syndrome
    C. trochanteric bursitis
    D. right sacroiliac joint problems

98. A physical therapist in a gait laboratory places a needle electrode in a calf muscle to record that muscle's activity during gait. The needle is inserted halfway down the calf and just behind the fibula. Which muscle is being tested?

    A. soleus
    B. flexor digitorum longus
    C. peroneus brevis
    D. flexor hallucis longus

99. A client fell and bruised the ischial tuberosity. Each of the following muscles has an attachment to the ischial tuberosity and thus could cause pain on contraction except:

    A. semitendinosus
    B. quadratus femoris
    C. gluteus minimus
    D. biceps femoris

100. A client injured the middle third of the sartorius muscle. The treatment intervention is to include phonophoresis and deep friction massage to the injured area. When applying any deep or penetrating treatment to the middle third of this muscle, it is important to remember that it overlies the adductor canal. The content of the adductor canal includes all of the following **except**:

    A. obturator nerve
    B. femoral artery
    C. saphenous nerve
    D. femoral vein

101. A therapist has been working with a client to increase gastrocnemius/soleus muscle strength. The muscle weakness is accompanied by numbness and tingling in the foot with no symptoms in the thigh or posterior calf. This would likely be a result of:

    A. peroneal nerve compression as it winds around the lateral malleolus
    B. tibia nerve compression in the tarsal tunnel
    C. compression of lateral plantar nerve in the heel region
    D. compression of medial plantar nerve in the heel region

102. Because dermatomal migration continues after myotomal migration is complete, loss of innervation to a muscle in one region results in loss of innervation to the skin in a region distal to the muscle. In order to recheck for a loss of muscle function after an intervention, which of the following could be done?

    A. For loss of peroneus tertius, test for cutaneous sensation over the first web space.
    B. For loss of peroneus longus, test for cutaneous sensation over the first through fourth toes, excluding the first web space.
    C. For loss of the vastus intermedius muscle, test for cutaneous sensation over the upper two thirds of the posterolateral leg.
    D. For loss of abductor hallucis brevis, test for cutaneous sensation over the medial surface of the foot.

103. A client has a movement dysfunction that includes limited ability to extend the knee and flex the thigh. The history includes a back strain injury just before the emergence of the weakness in the lower extremity. The treatment today will include PAs of:

    A. T-12
    B. L3
    C. L5
    D. S1-2

104. Strengthening exercises are being performed by a client with pes anserinus involvement. The three muscles that form the pes anserinus are:

    A. piriformis, psoas major, and psoas minor
    B. vastus medialis, vastus lateralis, and rectus femoris
    C. sartorius, gracilis, and semitendinosus
    D. sartorius, gracilis, and semimembranosus

105. **While attending a football game to observe a client recently discharged from physical therapy, you note that the client was tackled from the right while his RLE was firmly planted, placing his right knee in a valgus stress sufficient to tear the medial collateral ligament at the knee. What other structures were likely torn?**

    A. medial meniscus and posterior cruciate ligament (PCL)
    B. lateral meniscus and PCL
    C. lateral meniscus and anterior cruciate ligament (ACL)
    D. medial meniscus and ACL

106. **In order to strengthen the palmar interossei, treatment should focus on which of the following?**

    A. extension of the interphalangeal joints
    B. adduction of the fingers
    C. flexion of the metacarpophalangeal joints
    D. abduction of the fingers

107. **If a client's treatment program is designed to increase strength in order to perform functional activities involving lateral or external rotation of the shoulder, resistive exercises should focus on the:**

    A. infraspinatus
    B. deltoid
    C. latissimus dorsi
    D. supraspinatus

108. **A client with TBI is unable to depress the side of and retract his tongue. The primary muscles to be facilitated are the:**

    A. orbicularis oris and levator anguli oris
    B. hyoglossus and chondroglossus
    C. buccinator and masseter
    D. palatoglossus and palatopharyngeus

109. **Which muscle can be palpated starting at the anterior superior iliac spine and moving laterally along the iliac crest?**

    A. sartorius
    B. rectus femoris
    C. gluteus medius
    D. tensor fascia lata

110. **In distal segment fixed activities, right hip internal rotation is paired with which of the following?**

    A. left pelvis forward
    B. right pelvis forward
    C. left pelvis elevated
    D. left pelvis dropped

111. **In distal segment fixed activities, right hip internal rotation is paired with lumbar spine:**

    A. extension
    B. flexion
    C. rotation left
    D. rotation right

112. **A client underwent knee surgery (open joint, not arthroscopic). The surgery required more time than usual; however, a good result is expected. During evaluation, it is noted that the tourniquet may have been left on long enough to produce neuropraxis of the femoral nerve. This suspicion was confirmed regarding the neuropraxis, and the resultant weakness is a focus in the current treatment plan. The weakness observed involves the:**

    A. vastus lateralis and rectus femoris
    B. vastus medialis
    C. rectus femoris and vastus medialis
    D. vastus lateralis

113. Of the following definitions, which best describes skeletal muscle?

A. multinucleated, striated, and cylindrical
B. single nucleus, striated, and branched
C. multinucleated, striated, and fusiform
D. single nucleus, unstriated, and fusiform

114. The epithelium lining the trachea is:

A. simple squamous
B. stratified columnar
C. pseudostratified ciliated columnar
D. simple columnar with microvilli

115. Which is the correct ranking of tissues with regard to their ability to undergo repair? (The ranking is from high to low ability.)

A. articular cartilage, ligament, bone
B. ligament, bone, articular cartilage
C. bone, articular cartilage, ligament
D. bone, ligament, articular cartilage

116. The repair process in bone in response to fracture is an example of:

A. hypertrophy
B. hyperplasia
C. atrophy
D. necrosis

117. As part of treatment, a client is in a sidelying position and has been instructed to flex the hip to 90 degrees. That motion occurred around the _____ axis in the _____ plane.

A. anteroposterior/frontal
B. frontal/sagittal
C. longitudinal/transverse
D. horizontal/coronal

118. As the rate of loading increases, the stiffness of both bone and cartilage:

A. increases
B. decreases
C. does not change
D. decreases then increases

119. A client has been referred with a diagnosis of acquired immunodeficiency syndrome (AIDS) with decreased ability to perform ADLs. The client requires moderate assistance in all ADLs. The treatment today consists of transfer training and energy conservation techniques. The primary functional outcome of today's session is probably:

A. decreased energy expenditure
B. pain-free mobility
C. independence in transfers from bed to chair and chair to standing
D. independence in all aspects of ADLs with minimal energy expenditure

120. In documenting the progress that a client has made during today's treatment session, emphasis should be placed on:

A. level of strength, ROM, and endurance
B. short-term goal achievement expressed in functional outcomes
C. improvements since yesterday in ADLs
D. potential for accomplishing long-term goals

121. A physical therapist has reviewed the literature regarding the treatment of facet disorders in order to determine which technique has or techniques have been quantitatively researched and found to obtain the best results. This process of identifying the best is referred to as:

A. efficacy
B. effectiveness
C. efficiency
D. reliability

122. In reviewing an article in which two treatment procedures were compared, you note that a statistical difference was found. The level of significance identified by the authors was probably:

    A. $P > 1.0$
    B. $P > 0.05$
    C. $P < 0.05$
    D. $P < 0.25$

123. A research project that involves use of control groups and randomization is referred to as:

    A. descriptive
    B. experimental
    C. phenomenological
    D. quasi-experimental

124. Studies designed to discover the relationships and interactions among sociological, psychological, and educational variables are referred to as what kind of studies?

    A. descriptive
    B. anthropological
    C. field
    D. ethnographic

125. In a research project, when the numbers or symbols assigned to objects have no numerical meaning beyond the presence or absence of an attribute's being measured, the measurement is referred to as:

    A. ordinal
    B. nominal
    C. encoded
    D. inferential

126. In the _____ tests of significance, there is an estimation of at least one population parameter and there is an assumption that the findings can be generalized to the total population on the basis of the data.

    A. parametric
    B. nonparametric
    C. means comparison
    D. correlation

127. Chi-square data are commonly referred to as _____ statistics.

    A. parametric
    B. nonparametric
    C. means comparison
    D. correlation

128. The most commonly used statistical program used in qualitative studies is:

    A. Lotus
    B. Systat
    C. Mystat
    D. Statistical Package for Social Sciences

129. In measuring the differences between group means, the most commonly used test is:

    A. the t test
    B. the chi-square test
    C. the Wilcoxon test
    D. the Mann Whitney test

130. When looking at a series of individual comparisons in order to examine the differences among the groups, the test most commonly used is the:

    A. Wilcoxon sign
    B. multivariate analysis of variance (MANOVA)
    C. analysis of variance (ANOVA)
    D. Mann Whitney test

131. In a research project, the analysis of data includes more than one dependent variable. The test most commonly used in this situation is the:

    A. Wilcoxon sign
    B. MANOVA
    C. ANOVA
    D. Mann Whitney

132. Hypotheses are expected in which type of research?

    A. ethnographic
    B. phenomenological
    C. theoretical
    D. experimental

133. **In a client with AIDS, visual deficits are often caused by:**

    A. *Mycobacterium avium intracellulare*
    B. tuberculosis
    C. *Cytomegalovirus*
    D. thrush

134. **Treatment and goals for patients with cancer should focus on:**

    A. functional goals
    B. restoring normal ROM
    C. restoring strength to 5 on a scale of 5
    D. teaching the client transfer techniques

135. **An individual with a diagnosis of metastatic cancer who is undergoing chemotherapy may exhibit a decrease in platelet counts. This is referred to as:**

    A. leukopenia
    B. anemia
    C. thrombocytopenia
    D. pancytopenia

136. **Enlargement of lymph nodes without obvious pain is a classic symptom of:**

    A. Hodgkin's disease
    B. leukemia
    C. multiple myeloma
    D. thyroid cancer

137. **A client recently underwent colon surgery secondary to a new diagnosis of colon cancer. It is now 1 week after surgery, and the client is taking tube feedings and is resuming physical therapy. In which phase within the rehabilitation continuum is this client?**

    A. palliative
    B. restorative
    C. supportive
    D. communicative

138. **A client sustained severe burns over 30% of her body secondary to being struck by lightning. The tissue destruction extends to muscle, tendon, and bone. This burn would be referred to as:**

    A. superficial, partial thickness
    B. deep, partial thickness
    C. full thickness
    D. fourth-degree

139. **In the case of a full-thickness burn, it is consistent to find:**

    A. variable sensation in the wound bed
    B. rapid re-epithelialization from dermal elements
    C. re-epithelialization from the wound edges only
    D. risk of bacterial conversion

140. **An overgrowth of dermal elements with a thin, atrophic epidermis is a/an:**

    A. hypertrophic scar
    B. grade I ulceration
    C. normal scar tissue response
    D. reflective of decreased collagen synthesis

141. **A nonblanchable erythema of the skin is referred to as a:**

    A. hypertrophic scar
    B. grade I ulceration
    C. toxic epidermal necrolysis
    D. zone of stasis

142. **Using a whirlpool is contraindicated in the management of:**

    A. blood-borne pathogens
    B. absent pulses and deep tissue pain
    C. infected wounds
    D. dependent edema and venous congestion

143. **Ultrasonography is included in the care plan for a client with a non-healing wound. The rationale is that ultrasonography will:**

    A. increase collagen synthesis and improve tensile strength of tissue
    B. destroy *Staphylococcus aureus* bacteria
    C. increase capillary bed formation
    D. decrease pain

144. **The method of choice of treatment for venous insufficiency ulcers is use of:**

    A. an intermittent compression pump
    B. ultrasonography at 5 MHz
    C. active ROM exercises
    D. electrical stimulation

145. **Demonstrating unconditional positive regard to the client as a means of establishing rapport is referred to as:**

    A. sympathy
    B. interchangeable empathy
    C. empowerment
    D. behavior modification

146. **A hospice program worker is explaining the role of physical therapy to a group of family members. It is appropriate to include among the available services:**

    A. aggressive exercise programs
    B. teaching energy conservation techniques to the client
    C. prosthetic ordering and training
    D. passive range of motion (PROM) exercise programs

147. **The requirement to contact a payor before the provision of physical therapy services is:**

    A. a common requirement for therapists whose claims have been investigated
    B. to guarantee the client that appropriate services will be provided
    C. authorization
    D. capitation

148. **A 35-year-old permanently disabled client is being treated at home. The payor for the services will probably be under the _____ program.**

    A. Medicare
    B. Medicaid
    C. Veteran's Administration
    D. Americans with Disabilities

149. **Research studies have shown that the maximum penetration of topical agents via phonophoresis is:**

    A. < 0.5 inch
    B. > 0.5 inch
    C. < 0.5 cm
    D. > 5.0 cm

150. **The department administrator asks that two new high-level quadriplegics' programs be delegated to a new graduate physical therapist assistant. This request is declined, and the rationale is:**

    A. recent injuries and insecurities of the clients
    B. level of expertise required to perform treatments
    C. lack of experience of the assistant
    D. the therapist's desire to continue to treat these individuals

151. **Outriggers on an UE orthosis are designed to:**

    A. facilitate flexor strengthening
    B. increase ROM
    C. maintain and permit extension ROM
    D. approximate normal wrist and hand positioning

152. **The primary means for treating a client with a temporomandibular joint dysfunction involves:**

    A. relaxation and active ROM exercises
    B. superficial heat to reduce pain
    C. resistive exercises
    D. myofascial release techniques

153. **Which assistive device is most appropriate for gait training of a client who is a low-level (L4–5) paraplegic?**

    A. standard walker
    B. bilateral quadriped canes
    C. axillary crutches
    D. forearm crutches

154. **The most common bone malignancy in children is:**

    A. rhabdomyosarcoma
    B. synovial cell sarcoma
    C. liposarcoma
    D. osteosarcoma

155. **One of the social problems encountered by persons with a medical diagnosis of cancer is:**

    A. community rejection
    B. feelings of helplessness and hopelessness
    C. lower socioeconomic status
    D. societally limited resources

156. **Physical therapists in hospice programs assist clients in:**

    A. areas of mobility
    B. endurance development
    C. strengthening
    D. gait training

157. **A 10-year-old client was medically diagnosed as having acute lymphoblastic leukemia. The child has been hospitalized for medical management for 4 weeks and has decreased strength and endurance. The type of exercise program to implement is:**

    A. passive
    B. assistive
    C. active
    D. resistive

158. **A 15-year-old girl recently underwent an above-the-knee amputation secondary to a diagnosis of bone cancer. It is now 4 days after the amputation. The program to be implemented today is most likely:**

    A. residual limb conditioning
    B. bed mobility and transfer training
    C. gait training
    D. all of the above

159. **For the client in item 158, the psychosocial issues she is facing are:**

    A. rejection, fear, and depression
    B. anxiety, fear, and altered body image
    C. alienation, anxiety, and denial of her diagnosis
    D. altered body image, humiliation, and isolation

160. **A client had a pneumonectomy 5 days ago secondary to stage I lung cancer. This client was seen preoperatively and immediately postoperatively. The chest tubes have been removed. Today the client will be instructed in:**

    A. bed mobility and transfer training
    B. trunk mobility exercises
    C. coughing and shoulder AROM exercises
    D. deep breathing exercises

161. **In treating post-mastectomy clients, one of the most common problems is decreased mobility of the UE. Before starting a program of PROM or AROM exercises, it is important to make sure the tissue is pliable. To accomplish this, what should be used?**

    A. deep tissue friction massage
    B. ultrasonography
    C. iontophoresis
    D. effleurage and petrissage

162. **As a part of the treatment for a 40-year-old law enforcement officer who has radial nerve paresis secondary to a through-and-through gunshot wound, electrotherapy is being initiated today. The goal is to facilitate contractions of the musculature innervated by the radial nerve. The electrotherapy provides significant:**

    A. proprioceptive, kinesthetic, and cutaneous sensory input
    B. edema reduction in the wrist and hand
    C. strengthening of the involved musculature
    D. ROM retention

163. **If this is the first treatment session in which electrical stimulation will be used for a client who has a history of cardiac dysrhythmia, a primary precaution to be taken is to:**

    A. Keep the treatment time to a minimum.
    B. Only use low amperage and encourage the client to relax.
    C. Have electrocardiographic monitoring during the session.
    D. Use a very slow ramp time and continually seek feedback from the client.

164. **A client with chronic heart failure has been treated for 2 weeks. The care plan is focused on inspiratory muscle training (IMT). It would be consistent with current research findings to find:**

    A. no changes in maximal inspiratory pressure (MIP) and dyspnea
    B. improvements in MIP, maximal expiratory pressure (MEP), and dyspnea
    C. improvement in MIP but no change in MEP
    D. improvement in MIP and MEP but no change in dyspnea

165. **A 27-year-old electrical contractor is currently receiving an individualized home exercise program including Brandt/Daroff exercises for management of vertigo, which occurs whenever his neck is in extension. The symptoms have persisted for 12 years, and the medical diagnosis is benign paroxysmal positional vertigo (BPPV). Contemporary research findings indicate:**

    A. It is reasonable to expect complete resolution of symptoms, even after such a long history of dysfunction.
    B. Minimal improvement will occur, and the client will be able to assume the supine position without dizziness within 3 months.
    C. There will be no change in his symptoms, and treatment should be changed to either Epley or Semon approaches.
    D. Manual therapy intervention must be added to the program to achieve temporary resolution of symptoms.

166. **Of the following procedures, which has been used for edema reduction in clients with lymphedema?**

    A. cryotherapy
    B. phonophoresis
    C. whirlpool and Hubbard tank
    D. iontophoresis

167. **The electromotive force that determines the tendency of an electric charge to move, or an electric current to flow, from one point to another is referred to as:**

    A. action potential
    B. electrical potential
    C. afferent conduction
    D. efferent conduction

168. *Conduction velocity* is defined as:

A. an electrochemical event associated with the propagation of a wave of depolarization along the length of an excitable cell
B. the transmission of nerve impulses over motor nerves away from the central nervous system (CNS)
C. the speed with which a volley of nerve impulses travels along a bundle of nerve fibers
D. the speed of transmission of nerve impulses over sensory nerves toward the CNS

169. Two clients are being treated for peripheral nerve injuries. One is a neonate and the other is a 37-year-old carpenter. In reviewing the results of the nerve conduction velocity (NCV) studies, there is a substantial difference in the speed of transmission of nerve impulses. Which of the following differences can be expected?

A. slower conduction velocity in the neonate secondary to immaturity of the CNS
B. slower conduction velocity in the neonate secondary to the type of delivery, which resulted in a brachial plexus stretch injury
C. slower conduction velocity in the adult secondary to the normal aging process
D. slower conduction velocity in the adult secondary to the nature of his injury (i.e., excessive cervical extension)

170. The most common use for TENS is:

A. postsurgical pain
B. chronic LBP
C. pain related to bone cancers
D. acute LBP

171. An electrical engineer has been treated with TENS. The client asks how the TENS is able to reduce pain. The therapist's response is that the most prevalent (although highly criticized) theory, the Gate Control Theory of Pain Perception, is the best explanation at this time. The Gate Control Theory essentially says:

A. A reflex loop comes into play when electrical stimulation is applied to the area of greatest pain, which results in an analgesic effect.
B. The loss or diminishing of afferent input cancels the transmission of pain impulses from the spinal cord to the brainstem.
C. T cells transmit information along one or more of the ascending pathways to the centrally located thalamic and brainstem nuclei, which in turn release a hormone that in effect closes the gate to transmission of pain impulses.
D. TENS input is transmitted along large-diameter afferents, which in turn activate the inhibitory substantia gelatinosa (SG) interneurons, thus closing the gate to the transmission of nociceptive information.

172. Enkephalins, endorphins, serotonin, and dopamine operate in different parts of the CNS and are collectively referred to as:

A. endogenous opiates
B. healing hormones
C. chemicals released by the substantia gelatinosa
D. somatosensory signals

173. If a client is a candidate for superficial heat and the therapist wishes to combine it with active exercise of the wrist and hand, the modality of choice probably is:

A. paraffin bath
B. fluidotherapy
C. hydrocollator packs
D. infrared

174. **A client has a long history of ankle clonus. The therapist has decided to use cryotherapy in an attempt to reduce or eliminate the clonus. The modality that is supported by clinical research is:**

    A. cold packs
    B. ice massage
    C. cold whirlpool
    D. ice immersion

175. **Ultraviolet light treatment is being used for a client with psoriasis. Yesterday production of a minimal erythema dose (MED) occurred. Today a first-degree dose will be used. This is calculated as:**

    A. the time necessary to produce erythema
    B. 2.5 MED to produce erythema for up to 48 hours
    C. 5 MED to produce erythema and edema for up to 72 hours
    D. 10 MED to produce erythema and blistering

176. **A claims reviewer notes that the client received laser biostimulation. The purpose of the treatment was probably for:**

    A. reduction of LBP
    B. destruction of adhesions
    C. destruction of bacteria in an infected wound
    D. promotion of wound healing by optimizing scar formation

177. **When using a whirlpool bath to treat acute inflammation, the temperature of the water will probably be:**

    A. 50°F
    B. 70°F
    C. 90°F
    D. 100°F

178. **If aquatic therapy is to be used for a client who underwent a joint replacement, the exercise program will most likely be what kind of program?**

    A. deep water
    B. middle level to shallow level
    C. Bad Ragaz techniques
    D. aerobic

179. **CPM devices are commonly used in managing a number of different medical diagnoses. One of the primary benefits of CPM after ligament reconstruction is:**

    A. pain management
    B. reduction of edema
    C. reduction of adhesion formation
    D. prevention of atrophy

180. **Administration of intermittent compression (IC) to a client with UE edema has been delegated to an experienced physical therapist assistant. There are established parameters for UE and LE treatments. Which of the following pressure levels is appropriate for a client who demonstrates edema of the UE?**

    A. 20 to 50 mm Hg
    B. 30 to 70 mm Hg
    C. 40 to 80 mm Hg
    D. 50 to 90 mm Hg

181. **For the client in item 180, what might be a contraindication for IC?**

    A. infection
    B. altered cognitive state
    C. cardiac disease
    D. all of the above

182. **The client is 56 years old and has diabetes and coronary artery disease. The goal of an aerobic exercise program at this point is time is to:**

    A. improve functional ability level
    B. modify the risk factor of glucose intolerance
    C. condition the client overall before coronary artery bypass surgery (CABG)
    D. improve the client's self-image

183. **A client was referred with a diagnosis of angina pectoris. 63 years old and has a history of a progressively declining ability to ambulate. Could walk slowly only two to three blocks at a time before an episode of angina pectoris occurred. It was determined that the client was not a candidate for CABG because of triple vessel coronary artery disease. The left main artery was essentially clear, and the client had evidence of normal left ventricular function at rest. The type of program implemented for this client includes:**

    A. general warm-up exercises followed by walking up to his angina threshold
    B. general strengthening program and relaxation exercises
    C. high-impact aerobic exercises
    D. low-impact aerobic exercises

184. **The most common pulmonary emboli occur after:**

    A. CABG
    B. infectious pneumonia
    C. deep vein thrombosis in the LE
    D. a period of repeated asthma attacks

185. **The plan is to teach a client diaphragmatic breathing exercises today. The first step in the process is to:**

    A. Instruct the client to begin a series of slow, deep breaths and to concentrate on exhalation.
    B. Place the client's dominant hand over the mid–rectus abdominis area and his nondominant hand on the midsternal area.
    C. Direct the client to inhale slower through his mouth and try to increase the expansion of his chest every other breath.
    D. Apply firm counterpressure over the patient's mid–rectus abdominis area.

186. **The therapeutic objective of the diaphragmatic breathing exercise program is to:**

    A. improve oxygenation and ventilation
    B. decrease client dependence and depression
    C. alleviate dyspnea and improve the ease of breathing
    D. decrease respiratory rate

187. **In order to prevent dislodging of chest tubes in clients with lateral thoracotomies, the therapist should:**

    A. position the client on the non-operative side and avoid lateral rotation
    B. not abduct the shoulder on the side of the surgery more than 90 degrees
    C. position the client supine and avoid flexion and abduction beyond 90 degrees
    D. not flex the shoulder on the side of the surgery more than 80 degrees.

188. **In working with a client who is on bedrest for phlebitis, the ADL program should begin with:**

    A. rolling side to side at least every 2 hours
    B. UE strengthening and lower extremity AROM exercises
    C. long sitting general mobility exercises for the UEs
    D. reciprocal UE and LE AROM exercises

189. **The treatment emphasis for a client with atelectasis should include:**

    A. AROM of UEs and posture training to reduce kyphosis and musculoskeletal breathing limitations
    B. deep diaphragmatic breathing and postural drainage if secretions are present
    C. relaxation exercises and segmental breathing
    D. extended expiration and postural drainage

190. **A client is acutely ill and in the ICU secondary to hypoxia. The purpose of physical therapy at this point is to:**

    A. increase her vital capacity
    B. facilitate breathing by clearing her lungs
    C. decrease her fear and anxiety by teaching her to breathe calmly
    D. teach her techniques for conserving energy

191. **A client who is in the respiratory ICU begins to develop a dysrhythmia while being treated. The client is currently receiving 100% oxygen. What may have caused the dysrhythmia?**

    A. The client has a tracheal defect.
    B. The client may have experienced an anxiety attack.
    C. The exercise program may have been too vigorous.
    D. The suction catheter in the trachea caused vagal stimulation.

192. **What is a definite contraindication for postural drainage or pulmonary hygiene?**

    A. pneumonia
    B. cardiac tamponade
    C. osteoporosis
    D. pneumothorax

193. **One of the serious side effects of mechanical ventilation is:**

    A. increased risk of pulmonary infection
    B. inability to communicate
    C. psychological dependency
    D. inability to perform ADLs

194. **Of the four modes of mechanical ventilation, which one guarantees the client a predetermined number of mechanical breaths?**

    A. control
    B. assist
    C. assist-control
    D. intermittent mandatory ventilation

195. **Neonates compensate for respiratory difficulties by:**

    A. increasing the depth rather than the rate of ventilation
    B. increasing the rate rather than the depth of ventilation
    C. assuming a supine position
    D. assuming a prone position

196. **Which condition is commonly associated with the use of mechanical ventilation in premature infants?**

    A. pneumonia
    B. bronchopulmonary dysplasia
    C. decreased lung compliance
    D. respiratory failure

197. Monitoring for murmurs is essential when working with neonates. The murmur of a patent ductus arteriosus is usually characterized by:

A. a gurgling sound that also is associated with expiration
B. premature ventricular contractions that persist and accelerate during movement
C. increased blood pressure rate
D. short ejection murmur

198. A client reveals that spousal abuse has been occurring. The most appropriate action to be taken is to:

A. advise the client to seek professional help
B. discontinue any treatment that involves touching the client
C. document the statement and inform authorities
D. not react and to continue her treatment as planned

199. Before implementing treatment and conducting research, it is essential to obtain:

A. past medical records
B. the client's informed consent
C. authorization from the payor
D. the client's guarantee of payment for services

200. A client has received the maximum benefit from physical therapy. The administrator of the clinical practice requires that the client continue receiving services because the client's insurance plan permits six more visits. The proper course of action to be taken is to:

A. Discharge the client from physical therapy.
B. Contact the client's payor for clarification.
C. Find some other goal on which to work.
D. Resign and report the administrator.

Correct Responses to Sample Items in Chapter 4

1.	C	51.	B	101.	B	151.	C
2.	D	52.	C	102.	A	152.	A
3.	A	53.	B	103.	C	153.	D
4.	B	54.	C	104.	C	154.	D
5.	C	55.	B	105.	D	155.	C
6.	B	56.	A	106.	B	156.	A
7.	A	57.	D	107.	A	157.	C
8.	D	58.	B	108.	B	158.	D
9.	C	59.	D	109.	D	159.	B
10.	B	60.	A	110.	A	160.	B
11.	C	61.	C	111.	C	161.	A
12.	B	62.	B	112.	B	162.	A
13.	C	63.	A	113.	A	163.	C
14.	A	64.	D	114.	C	164.	B
15.	C	65.	A	115.	D	165.	A
16.	C	66.	B	116.	B	166.	D
17.	B	67.	C	117.	B	167.	B
18.	D	68.	C	118.	A	168.	C
19.	B	69.	D	119.	C	169.	A
20.	A	70.	B	120.	B	170.	B
21.	C	71.	B	121.	A	171.	D
22.	D	72.	A	122.	B	172.	A
23.	B	73.	D	123.	D	173.	B
24.	A	74.	C	124.	C	174.	C
25.	B	75.	B	125.	B	175.	B
26.	B	76.	A	126.	A	176.	D
27.	C	77.	D	127.	B	177.	A
28.	B	78.	A	128.	D	178.	B
29.	D	79.	D	129.	A	179.	C
30.	A	80.	C	130.	C	180.	A
31.	B	81.	D	131.	B	181.	D
32.	A	82.	A	132.	D	182.	B
33.	C	83.	C	133.	C	183.	A
34.	D	84.	B	134.	A	184.	C
35.	B	85.	B	135.	C	185.	B
36.	B	86.	D	136.	A	186.	C
37.	A	87.	A	137.	B	187.	D
38.	C	88.	C	138.	D	188.	A
39.	D	89.	B	139.	C	189.	B
40.	B	90.	A	140.	A	190.	B
41.	D	91.	B	141.	B	191.	D
42.	A	92.	C	142.	D	192.	C
43.	C	93.	A	143.	C	193.	A
44.	B	94.	B	144.	A	194.	A
45.	D	95.	D	145.	B	195.	B
46.	A	96.	A	146.	B	196.	B
47.	D	97.	B	147.	C	197.	D
48.	A	98.	D	148.	A	198.	C
49.	B	99.	C	149.	A	199.	B
50.	C	100.	A	150.	B	200.	A

References

All of the references identified in Chapters 2 and 3 are relevant to this chapter. Additionally, the following references were used and are recommended for reading:

Almeida, GL, Campbell, SR, Girolami, GL, et al.: Multidimensional assessment of motor function in a child with cerebral palsy following intrathecal administration of baclofen. Phys Ther 1997, 77:751–764.

Cahalin, LP, Simigran, MJ, and Dec, GW: Inspiratory muscle training in patients with chronic heart failure awaiting cardiac transplantation: Results of a pilot clinical trial. Phys Ther 1997, 77:830–838.

Ford-Smith, CD: The individualized treatment of a patient with benign paroxysmal positional vertigo. Phys Ther 1997, 77:848–855.

Irwin, S, and Tecklin, JS (eds): Cardiopulmonary Physical Therapy. St. Louis, The C.V. Mosby Company, 1990.

Knuttsson, E, and Mattssan, E: Effects of local cooling on monosynaptic reflexes in man. Scan J Rehabil Med 1969, 1:126–140.

McGarvey, CL (ed): Physical Therapy for the Cancer Patient. New York, Churchill Livingstone, 1990.

Michlovitz, SL: Cryotherapy. In Michlovitz, SL (ed): Thermal Agents in Rehabilitation, ed 2. Philadelphia, FA Davis Company, 1996.

Miglietta, O: Action of cold on spasticity. Am J Phys Med 1973, 52:198–213.

Miglietta, O: Electromyographic characteristics of clonus and influence of cold. Arch Phys Med Rehabil 1964, 45:508–515.

Monteiro, ME: Physical therapy implications following the TRAM procedure. Phys Ther 1997, 77:765–770.

Roach, KE, Brown, MD, Albin, RD, et al.: The sensitivity and specificity of pain response to activity and position in categorizing patients with low back pain. Phys Ther 1997, 77:730–738.

Smith, TL, et al.: New skeletal muscle model for the longitudinal study of alterations in microcirculation following contusion and cryotherapy. Microsurgery 1993, 14:487–499.

Wolf, SL (ed): Electrotherapy. New York, Churchill Livingstone, 1981.

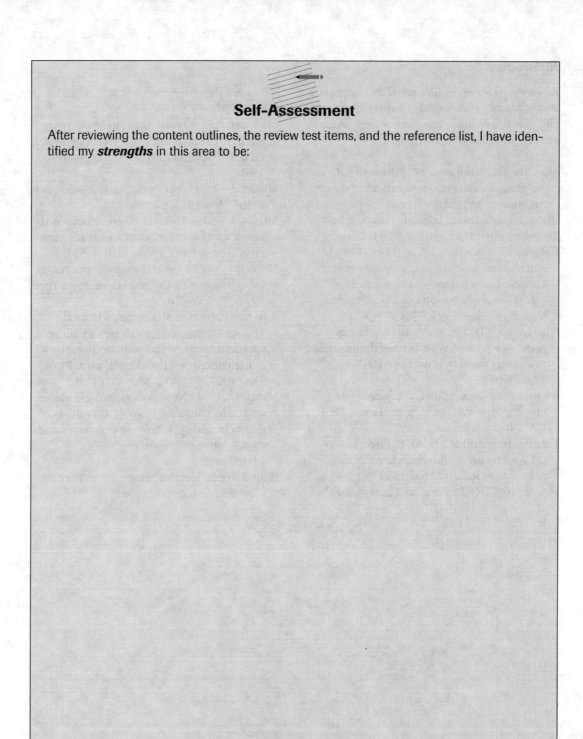

Self-Assessment

After reviewing the content outlines, the review test items, and the reference list, I have identified my *strengths* in this area to be:

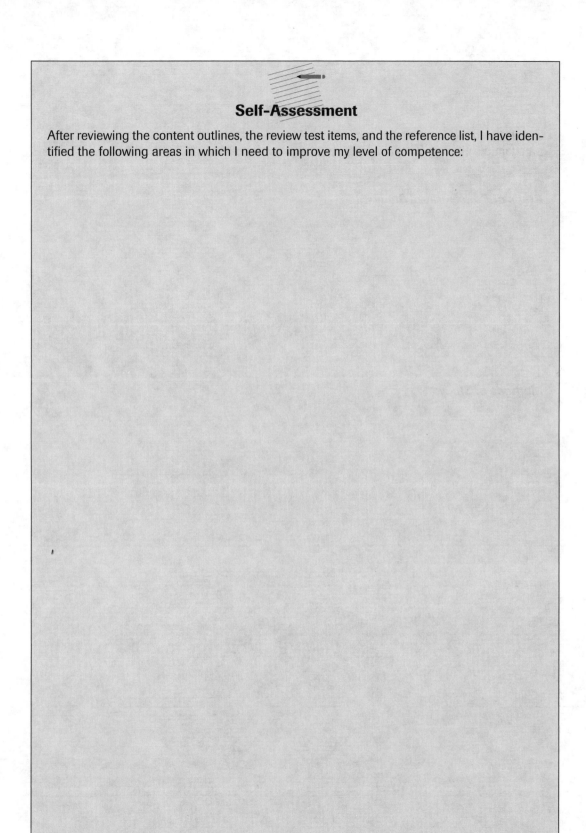

Self-Assessment

After reviewing the content outlines, the review test items, and the reference list, I have identified the following areas in which I need to improve my level of competence:

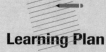

Learning Plan

In order to improve my level of competence, I have identified the following areas of concentrated study, the method(s) by which I will study, and the timelines for each area:

Areas of Concentrated Study:

Methods of Study:

Timelines:

Notes

Appendix A
State Boards of Physical Therapy

The following are the state boards that have the responsibility and authority to license physical therapists. Detailed information regarding the practice acts and requirements is available from each legal jurisdiction as well as the APTA *State Licensure Reference Guide,* which is published annually. The sources of the information included in this Appendix are the individual state boards and the *State Licensure Reference Guide 1997,* which is published annually by the American Physical Therapy Association.

Legal Jurisdiction	Agency Name	Address	Telephone	FAX
Alabama	Alabama Board of Physical Therapy	400 S. Union Street Suite 315 Montgomery, AL 36104	(334) 242-4064	(334) 240-3288
Alaska	State Physical Therapy & Occupational Therapy Board Dept of Commerce & Economic Development	P.O. Box 110806 Juneau, AK 99811-0806	(907) 465-2551	(907) 465-2974
Arizona	Arizona State Board of Physical Therapy Examiners	1400 W. Washington Suite 230 Phoenix, AZ 85007	(602) 542-3095	(602) 542-3093
Arkansas	Arkansas State Board of Physical Therapy	Three Financial Centre Suite 300 900 S. Shackleford Little Rock, AR 72211	(501) 228-7100	(501) 228-5535
California	State Board of Physical Therapy	1434 Howe Avenue Suite 92 Sacramento, CA 95825	(916) 263-2550	(916) 263-2560
Colorado	Physical Therapy Licensure	1560 Broadway Suite 680 Denver, CO 80202	(303) 894-2440	Not available
District of Columbia	D.C. Board of Physical Therapy Dept of Consumer or Regulatory Affairs Occupation and Professional Licensing Administration	614 H Street, NW Ninth Floor, Room 923 Washington, DC 20001	(202) 727-7465	(202) 727-7662
Florida	Agency for Health Care Administration	1940 N. Monroe Street Tallahassee, FL 32399-0789	(904) 487-3372	(904) 921-7865
Georgia	Georgia State Board of Physical Therapy State Examining Boards	166 Pryor Street, SW Atlanta, GA 30303	(404) 656-3921	(404) 651-9532
Hawaii	Dept of Commerce & Consumer Affairs Professional & Vocational Licensing Div. Board of Physical Therapy	1010 Richards Street P.O. Box 3469 Honolulu, HI 96801	(808) 586-3000	Not available
Idaho	Idaho Board of Medicine	280 N. 8th Street, Suite 202 P.O. Box 83720 Boise, ID 83720-0058	(208) 334-2822	(208) 334-2801

Continued on page 128

Legal Jurisdiction	Agency Name	Address	Telephone	FAX
Illinois	Dept of Professional Regulation	320 W. Washington 3rd Floor Springfield, IL 62786	(217) 782-8556	(217) 782-7645
Indiana	Health Professions Bureau	402 W. Washington Room 041 Indianapolis, IN 46204	(317) 232-2960	(317) 233-4236
Iowa	Dept of Public Health/ Bureau of Professional Licensure Board of Physical Therapy & Occupational Therapy Examiners	Lucas Building, 4th Floor Des Moines, IA 50319-0075	(515) 281-7074	(515) 281-3121
Kansas	Kansas State Board of Healing Arts	235 S.W. Topeka Boulevard Topeka, KS 66603	(913) 296-7413	(913) 296-0852
Kentucky	Kentucky State Board of Physical Therapy	9110 Leesgate Road, #6 Louisville, KY 40222-5159	(502) 595-4687	(502) 595-4687
Louisiana	Louisiana State Board of Physical Therapy Examiners	2014 W. Pinhook, #701 Lafayette, LA 70508	(318) 262-1043	(318) 262-1054
Maine	Board of Examiners in Physical Therapy Dept of Professional & Financial Regulation	State House Station, #35 Augusta, ME 04333	(207) 624-8603	(207) 624-8637
Maryland	Board of Physical Therapy Examiners	4201 Patterson Avenue, #318 Baltimore, MD 21215-2299	(410) 764-4752	(410) 358-1183
Massachusetts	Board of Allied Health	100 Cambridge Street Room 1516 Boston, MA 02202	(800) 359-1313, Applications: (617) 727-3071	(617) 727-2197
Michigan	Department of Commerce	BOPR/Health Services P.O. Box 30018 Lansing, MI 48909	(517) 373-3596	(517) 373-2179
Minnesota	Board of Medical Practice Physical Therapy Advisory Council	2700 University Avenue West, Suite 106 St. Paul, MN 55114-1080	(612) 642-00538	(612) 642-0393
Mississippi	Mississippi State Department of Health Professional Licensure	P.O. Box 1700 Jackson, MS 39215-1700	(601) 987-4153	(601) 987-3784
Missouri	Missouri Board of Healing Arts	P.O. Box 4 Jefferson City, MO 65102	(573) 751-0144	(573) 751-3166
Montana	Department of Commerce Division of Public Safety Board of Physical Therapy Examiners	111 N. Jackson P.O. Box 200513 Helena, MT 59620-0513	(406) 444-3728	(406) 444-1667
Nebraska	Department of Health, Professional and Occupational Licensure Division	301 Centennial Mall South P.O. Box 95007 Lincoln, NE 68509-5007	(402) 471-2299	(402) 471-3577

Continued on page 129

Legal Jurisdiction	Agency Name	Address	Telephone	FAX
Nevada	Nevada State Board of Physical Therapy Examiners	P.O. Box 81467 Las Vegas, NV 89180-1467	(702) 876-5535	(702) 876-2097
New Hampshire	Board of Registration in Medicine	2 Industrial Park Drive Concord, NH 03301	(603) 271-1203	(603) 271-6702
New Jersey	New Jersey State Board of Physical Therapy	124 Halsey Street, 6th Floor P.O. Box 45014 Newark, NJ 07101	(201) 504-6455	None
New Mexico	New Mexico Physical Therapists' Licensing Board	P.O. Box 25101 725 St. Michael's Drive Santa Fe, NM 87504	(505) 827-7162	(505) 827-7095
New York	State Board for Physical Therapy State Education Department	Cultural Education Center Room 3019 Albany, NY 12230	(518) 474-6374	(518) 473-6995
North Carolina	North Carolina Board of Physical Therapy Examiners	18 W. Colony Place Suite 120 Durham, NC 27705	(919) 490-6393	(919) 490-5106
North Dakota	North Dakota State Examining Committee for Physical Therapists	Box 69 Grafton, ND 58237	(701) 352-0125	(701) 352-3093
Ohio	Ohio Occupational Therapy, Physical Therapy, and Athletic Trainers Board	77 S. High Street 16th Floor Columbus, OH 43266-0317	(614) 466-3774	(614) 644-8112
Oklahoma	Oklahoma State Board of Medical Licensure and Supervision	5104 N. Francis, Suite C OR P.O. Box 18256 Oklahoma City, OK 73154	(405) 848-6841	(405) 848-8240
Oregon	Oregon Physical Therapist Licensing Board	800 NE Oregon Avenue Suite 407 Portland, OR 97232	(503) 731-4047	None
Pennsylvania	Pennsylvania State Board of Physical Therapy	P.O. Box 2649 Harrisburg, PA 17105-2649	(717) 783-7134	(717) 787-7769
Puerto Rico	Office of Regulation and Certification of the Professions of Health	Call Box 10200 Santurce, PR 00908-0200	(809) 725-8161, Ext. 209	(809) 725-7903
Rhode Island	Rhode Island Board of Examiners in Physical Therapy	Three Capitol Hill 104 Cannon Building Providence, RI 02908-5097	(401) 277-2827	(401) 277-1272
South Carolina	State Board of Physical Therapy Examiners	3600 Forest Drive P.O. Box 11329 Columbia, SC 29211-1329	(803) 734-4170	(803) 734-4218
South Dakota	South Dakota State Board of Medical & Osteopathic Examiners	1323 S. Minnesota Avenue Sioux Falls, SC 57105	(605) 334-8343	(605) 336-0270
Tennessee	Tennessee Board of Occupational Therapy and Physical Therapy	283 Plus Park Boulevard Nashville, TN 37247-1010	(423) 392-7053	(423) 393-7055

Continued on page 130

Legal Jurisdiction	Agency Name	Address	Telephone	FAX
Texas	Texas State Board of Physical Therapy Examiners	333 Guadeloupe, Suite 2-510 Austin, TX 78701	(512) 305-6900	(512) 305-6970
Utah	Division of Occupational and Professional Licensing	160 East 300 South P.O. Box 45805 Salt Lake City, UT 84145-0802	(801) 530-6767	(801) 530-6511
Vermont	Office of Professional Regulation Office of Secretary of State Licensing and Registration Division	109 State Street Montpelier, VT 05609-1106	(802) 828-2390	(802) 2496
Virginia	Department of Health Professions Board of Medicine	6606 W. Broad Street 4th Floor Richmond, VA 23230-1717	(804) 662-9073	(804) 662-9943
Virgin Islands	Virgin Islands Board of Physical Therapy Examiners Department of Health	48 Sugar Estate St. Thomas, VI 00802	(809) 776-8311	(809) 777-4001
Washington	Department of Health	1300 SE Quince Street P.O. Box 47868 Olympia, WA 98504-7868	(360) 753-3132, General Information; (360) 753-0876, Applications	(360) 753-0657
West Virginia	West Virginia Board of Physical Therapy	Route 1, Box 306 Lost Creek, WV 26385	(304) 745-4161	(304) 745-4165
Wisconsin	Department of Regulation and Licensing Medical Examining Board	P.O. Box 8935 Madison, WI 53708	(608) 267-9377	(608) 267-0644
Wyoming	Wyoming State Board of Physical Therapy	2020 Carey Avenue Suite 201 Cheyenne, WY 82002	(307) 777-6529	(307) 777-3508

Because of the differences in state requirements and processes, you should contact the specific agency for the jurisdiction in which you wish to practice. An excellent overall reference for the state boards is the annually published APTA *Statement Licensure Reference Guide.* You may contact the APTA at (800) 999-APTA for information regarding cost and purchase of the guide.

Appendix B
Glossary of Terms

In every country there are terms that are unique to the language(s) of that country and the historical development of usage. The purpose of this appendix is to identify commonly used terms that may be unique to practice in the United States, its territories, and the District of Columbia. It is not an exhaustive list, but one that may help you as you study for the licensure examination. For the most part, the list consists of abbreviations.

1.	a	before
2.	AFO	ankle fixed orthosis. This was previously referred to as a *short leg brace;* it prevents ankle movement
3.	AK	above-the-knee, as in amputation
4.	BK	below the knee
5.	c	with
6.	C/O or c/o	complains of
7.	Dx	diagnosis
8.	ENMG	electroneuromyography
9.	forearm crutches	These were previously referred as *Lofstrands.*
10.	FWB	full weight bearing as applied to gait or ambulation
11	GSW	gun shot wound
12.	NDT	neurodevelopmental techniques, also referred to as *Bobath*
13.	neonate	newborn infant
14.	p	after or following
15.	p1	refers to where pain starts or is first present
16.	p2	refers to where pain ends
17.	Plinth	treatment table
18.	pt.	patient or client
19.	PT	physical therapist
20.	PTA	physical therapist assistant
21.	PTB	patellar tendon bearing; refers to a prosthesis
22.	PWB	partial weight bearing as applied to gait or ambulation
23.	R/O	rule out, as in rule out one diagnosis in light of findings
24.	Rx	treatment
25.	s	without
26.	sx	symptoms
27.	T&T	through and through
28.	Tx	traction
29.	w/c	wheelchair
30.	<	less than
31.	>	greater than
32.	//	parallel bars
33.	↺	rotation to the left; commonly used in manual therapy when referring to the trunk
34.	↻	rotation to the right; commonly used in manual therapy when referring to the trunk
35.	✔	flexion

It is strongly recommended that you acquire a medical terminology text or programmed instruction book that has been published in the United States in order to ensure your understanding, translation, and comprehension of medical terminology as used by physical therapists in the United States.

For individuals educated in the United States, it is highly recommended that you review a medical terminology text and other national references to ensure that you are using terminology and symbols accepted by the various components of the healthcare delivery system, including third party payors, governmental agencies, and the community of practitioners and scholars in physical therapy.

Appendix C
Comprehensive Multiple Choice Examination for Physical Therapists

The licensure examination is now offered on computer. A touch screen or scrolling allows the test taker to move through the items and select the correct responses. Remember that more than one answer may seem possible or may actually be true. What determines the correct answer may be a hierarchy, for example, sequential steps in a process; may involve a more specific answer; or may require a broader more encompassing response. If in doubt, the item may be flagged and returned to later. There is no harm in guessing because only correct responses are counted. For purposes of the study examination, it is suggested that an answer sheet be prepared to indicate choices and, if in doubt, which choices may be correct. Continue all the way through the examination and then recheck only those items for which there was some doubt, make a selection, and complete the examination. When finished, check the answers against the correct responses, which are contained in Appendix E. Good luck.

1. **A physiological or accessory movement:**

   A. can exceed the anatomical limit of a motion
   B. can be performed within the pathological limit of motion
   C. cannot be performed beyond the pathological limit
   D. can be performed in all fibrous joints

2. **According to contemporary research on the clinical reliability of manual muscle testing (MMT):**

   A. MMT has poor inter-tester reliability on grades below Fair.
   B. Staff physical therapists can perform MMT reliably in a clinical setting.
   C. Physical therapists are reliable with one half a grade.
   D. Using dynamometers is not any more reliable than using MMT.

3. **A construction worker complains of pain in his left knee after standing all day. To relieve this pain, the leg must be elevated for 1 hour before it goes away. What information indicates severity?**

   A. Elevation of the foot is required to relieve pain.
   B. There is pain in the left knee.
   C. The client is a construction worker.
   D. The client's occupation requires standing all day at work.

4. **A 14-year-old comes to the clinic complaining of pain on the bottom of the heel of the left lower extremity (LLE) when playing basketball. The client was recently selected to participate on two teams and plays basketball 6 days a week for at least 1 to 2 hours a day. On examination, pain is experienced when the lateral edges of the heel are squeezed. The nature of the problem is most likely:**

   A. Achilles tendinitis
   B. Sever's disease
   C. Achilles bursitis
   D. calcaneal stress fracture

5. **Which one of the following statements is true about a capsular pattern of ROM limitation?**

   A. It does not involve a fixed number of degrees for each motion, but rather, a fixed proportion of one motion relative to another motion.
   B. It is usually caused by a condition involving structures such as ligament shortening, muscle strains, or muscle contractures.
   C. It usually involves only one or two motions of a joint in contrast to non-capsular patterns, which involve all or most motions of a joint.
   D. Joints in which their movements have more firm end feels tend to develop capsular patterns.

6. A 27-year-old client reports finding enlarged axillary and cervical lymph nodes beginning over 1 month ago. Also presents with a fever and complains of fatigue and weight loss. Questioning and physical examination reveal no evidence of joint pain or visible skin changes. At this point in the assessment, the appropriate action is to:

   A. Continue with a more extensive objective evaluation.
   B. Refer to the client's primary care physician.
   C. Begin a treatment program of active range-of-motion (AROM) and active-assisted range-of-motion (AAROM) exercises.
   D. Include cryotherapy as a part of treatment approach.

7. A soccer player is being evaluated and reports pain in the anterior compartment muscles that began with pain at heel strike and has progressed to the point of the client's being unable to hold the forefoot up during foot descent and eccentric contractions. The diagnosis suspected is:

   A. stress fractures
   B. shin splints
   C. tendonitis
   D. myositis

8. In examining a client who reports joint pain, "ballotting" the joint is performed to:

   A. determine the passive range of motion (PROM)
   B. elicit the presence of fluid
   C. assess for increased heat over the joint
   D. determine the presence of crepitus

9. Which one of the following is a normal response to exercise exhibited by blood pressure?

   A. Systolic pressure remains the same during active exercise.
   B. Systolic pressure returns to the normal resting value 15 to 20 minutes after exercising
   C. Systolic pressure gradually increases with exercise and plateaus as the exercise intensity plateaus, and declines as exercise intensity declines.
   D. Diastolic pressure increases more than 10 to 15 mm Hg during the exercise or activity.

10. During the chart review of a patient with insulin-dependent diabetes mellitus referred for evaluation, it is normal to expect to find abnormally high amounts of which of the following substances in the blood?

    A. lipids
    B. cholesterol
    C. glucose
    D. all of the above

11. What type of contraction occurs when the force of a muscle is less than the resistance?

    A. concentric
    B. eccentric
    C. isometric
    D. isokinetic

12. A new patient has a diagnosis of poliomyelitis. Which of the following will be found on evaluation?

    A. hyperactive deep tendon reflexes
    B. spotty sensory deficits
    C. spotty muscle weakness
    D. paresthesia of affected extremities

13. A shoulder quadrant test should be performed:

    A. every time passive mobility testing for the shoulder is done
    B. if the patient has no pain on other passive mobility tests
    C. to assess for laxity in a patient with chronic shoulder pain
    D. if the patient has pain on passive glenohumeral flexion or abduction

14. **A 20-year-old collegiate swimmer presents with left anterior shoulder pain. The client swims freestyle and experiences increased pain as the arm is raised above the head and enters the water. The client is unable to lie on the left shoulder or abduct through an arc of 90 to 120 degrees without pain. The greatest pain occurs with a combination of end-range flexion with internal rotation. These findings are consistent with:**

   A. posterior shoulder instability
   B. acromioclavicular (AC) joint arthritis
   C. rotator cuff strain
   D. impingement

15. **A patient complains of dizziness when looking over the right shoulder while backing the car out of the driveway. Vertebral artery testing:**

   A. should be done if the intent is to perform a G.II to the cervical spine
   B. results would be positive if the patient had a symptom of facial paresthesia
   C. would be performed if the patient had PROM of cervical rotation of 30 degrees right
   D. would only be indicated if the patient also complains of dizziness with other activities that involve cervical rotation

16. **The typical presentation of carpal tunnel syndrome may include all of the following except:**

   A. awakening at night because of fourth and fifth digit pain or tingling
   B. atrophy of the thenar eminence
   C. wrist and hand pain
   D. higher incidence with pregnancy

17. **A client was evaluated for left hemiplegia and demonstrated rehabilitation potential. The goals for this client should focus on:**

   A. the levels of services where treatment will be provided
   B. the client's goals
   C. functional outcomes that are likely to be achieved
   D. falling within the parameters delineated by the payor

18. **The advantage of performing a myelogram over a plain radiography is that:**

   A. a myelogram allows direct visualization of the spinal cord, but a radiogram does not.
   B. a myelogram allows visualization of the thecal (dural) sac, but a radiogram does not.
   C. a myelogram allows visualization of all surrounding soft tissues, but a radiogram does not.
   D. a myelogram shows areas of increased cellular activity indicating areas of inflammation, but a radiogram does not.

19. **A 27-year-old client complains of night pain in both wrists and paresthesias along the volar aspect of the thumb and index, middle, and half of the ring fingers. Which orthotic device is most appropriate?**

   A. a pneumatic cuff
   B. a long arm splint with the elbow flexed less than 90 degrees
   C. a hand-based thumb spica splint
   D. a wrist extension splint with the wrist in 20 to 30 degrees extension
   E. a wrist splint with the wrist in the neutral position

20. **A client presents with a diagnosis of thoracic outlet syndrome (TOS). To rule out cervical nerve root involvement, which of the following tests are indicated?**

   A. Roos test
   B. slump test
   C. Adson's test
   D. foraminal compression test

21. **A professional golfer is referred for evaluation and treatment. The referral indicates that the client is 6 weeks post–right elbow fracture. During the evaluation, it is determined that the client is lacking 20 degrees of extension with PROM. Which of the following would probably increase the elbow extension ROM?**

   A. posterior to anterior (PA) of the radial head on the humerus
   B. PA of the radial head on the ulna
   C. anterior to posterior (AP) of the coronoid process
   D. distraction of the ulna

22. **TOS can result from which of the following?**

   A. a cervical rib
   B. a large callous from a healed clavicular fracture
   C. prolonged overhead work
   D. all of the above

23. **One of the tests used in assessing a neonate is to assess the rooting reflex. This test is administered by:**

   A. stroking the upper lip and waiting for the lip to retract
   B. using a finger to lightly stroke the corner of the infant's mouth
   C. using a finger to firmly apply pressure to the corner of the infant's mouth
   D. any of the above

24. **A 23-year-old man suffered a spinal cord injury (SCI) while rock climbing. The client is independent in transfers, which indicates that the cord level involved is below:**

   A. C5
   B. C6
   C. C7
   D. T1

25. **A 35-year-old woman is referred by a rheumatologist for evaluation and treatment. She had consulted with a variety of physicians without a diagnosis until she was examined by the rheumatologist. The medical diagnosis is fibromyalgia. Based on this information, it can be predicted that the client most likely:**

   A. is very satisfied with the healthcare system
   B. will focus the dialogue on anything but her symptoms
   C. has issues similar to persons with disabilities after primary neurological disorders
   D. will appreciate your validation when you describe her condition as psychosomatic

26. **The main problem for a 70-year-old client with Parkinson's disease could be expected to include all of the following except:**

   A. decreased balance
   B. bradykinesia
   C. kyphotic posture
   D. hypotonicity

27. **When performing a subjective evaluation of an 82-year-old client who is in acute inpatient care secondary to a right cerebrovascular accident (CVA), it is important to:**

   A. get information from the chart only because the patient may be unreliable
   B. allow the patient time to respond because cognitive processing may be slowed
   C. defer obtaining information pertaining to the home environment because you do not want to give the patient false hope
   D. develop the subjective portion of the examination thoroughly and completely before beginning the objective examination

28. During a home health visit, it is noted that an 80-year-old client is edematous, has flaky skin and a protruding abdomen, and is very apathetic. A cause of these symptoms may be:

A. vitamin C deficiency
B. vitamin D overabundance
C. kwashiorkor
D. Ca^{++} deficiency

29. A 60-year-old client complains of back pain after performing certain movements during the evaluation. Which of the following subjective complaints is most indicative of an osteoporotic fracture?

A. The client complains of unilateral pain radiating into the buttock and leg.
B. The client states that pain is constant and not relieved by changing positions.
C. The client states that forward flexion of the trunk reduces her pain.
D. The client states that there was no trauma before the onset of back pain.

30. Ankylosing spondylitis is a disease that can be difficult to diagnose because:

A. It has an insidious onset.
B. The symptoms may be mild and non-progressive.
C. The symptoms can be confused with mechanical low back dysfunction.
D. All of the above

31. A client currently receiving therapy presents with pitting edema of both feet. This may be a sign of:

A. cor pulmonale
B. pneumonia
C. atelectasis
D. excessive activity

32. An advantage of a tracheostomy in a ventilator-dependent patient is that it:

A. increases the dead air space
B. increases the residual volume
C. allows the patient to eat
D. all of the above

33. A client has been seen for 3 days. When the therapist enters the client's room, the client is found lying in bed. The client's respiratory rate is 40 breaths per minute; there is left ankle and leg edema with a positive Homan's sign; and the body temperature is 98.6°F. Given the following choices, the most likely cause of tachypnea is:

A. cor pulmonale
B. pulmonary embolus
C. pneumonia
D. emphysema

34. When assessing a client's respiratory rate:

A. It may be measured by placing a hand on the client's diaphragm and ribcage.
B. It may be measured for 10 seconds.
C. It should be taken only after the patient is fully informed of what is being done.
D. It may be measured by placing a hand on the lateral aspect of the last two ribs.

35. The study of motion regardless of the forces that produce it is a definition of:

A. kinetics
B. kinematics
C. dynamics
D. statics

36. The tibialis anterior functions as what class of lever during a concentric contraction in an open kinematic chain?

A. first
B. second
C. third
D. fourth

37. In which lever system does the effort force always have the greatest mechanical advantage?

A. first
B. second
C. third
D. fourth

38. **In articular cartilage, which zone has the greatest porosity?**

   A. superficial tangential
   B. middle
   C. deep
   D. subcontral

39. **Which of the following provides both mechanical strength and a diffusion barrier to the axons it surrounds?**

   A. epimysium
   B. perimysium
   C. endomysium
   D. none of the above

40. **Which type of contraction occurs in which the origins and insertions of the contracting muscles are brought closer together because of the action of the muscle?**

   A. concentric
   B. eccentric
   C. isometric
   D. isokinetic

41. **In a concentric contraction, velocity is _____ related to load.**

   A. directly
   B. inversely
   C. never
   D. maximally

42. **In which structure(s) is the vestibular nucleus located?**

   A. medulla
   B. pons
   C. midbrain
   D. medulla and pons

43. **The part of the primary motor cortex that controls movement of the thigh is supplied by which of the following arteries?**

   A. anterior cerebral
   B. middle cerebral
   C. posterior cerebral
   D. anterior and middle cerebral

44. **In the brainstem, the _____ _____ links cranial nerve nuclei that control extraocular muscles with the vestibular nucleus.**

   A. medial vestibulospinal tract
   B. lateral lemniscus
   C. medial lemniscus
   D. lateral vestibulospinal tract

45. **A lesion in the left area 19 of the brain could result in an inability to recognize:**

   A. voices
   B. tactile stimuli
   C. written words
   D. melodies

46. **Which of the following is not likely to affect a person's short-term performance?**

   A. medications he or she is taking on a regular basis
   B. distractions present in the environment
   C. the amount of fatigue he or she has from continuously practicing the task
   D. a lack of interest in the activity he or she is performing

47. **With a client who presents with weakness of the left extensor carpi radialis, you choose to use electrical stimulation as a part of your evaluation. Of the following choices, which one has been shown to stimulate the most forceful contractions?**

   A. beat-modulated alternating current (AC)
   B. straight, unmodulated AC
   C. monophasic pulsatile current
   D. biphasic symmetrical pulsatile current

48. **For the client described in item 47, it would be most appropriate and most likely necessary to examine which of the following extents in your objective examination?**

   A. short of provoking low back pain (LBP) and buttock pain
   B. to the limit of AROM or PROM that produces LBP and buttock pain
   C. to the end of the available AROM or PROM plus overpressure
   D. to the point of provoking LE pain

49. Gristly, elastic connective tissue composed of specialized cells in a translucent, pearly-blue matrix is the definition of:

A. hyaline cartilage
B. ligamentous structures
C. white fibrocartilage
D. bipennate muscle fibers

50. Which disease is a recessive genetic metabolic disorder characterized by pellagra-like skin lesions, transient cerebellar ataxia, and hyper-aminoaciduria?

A. Hashimoto's disease
B. Hartnup disease
C. Hansen's disease
D. Hers' disease

51. The F wave recorded in electroneu-romyographic testing appears on _____ stimulation of a motor nerve and is caused by an-tidromic transmission of a stimulus.

A. submaximal
B. supramaximal
C. subminimal
D. minimal

52. An area on the surface of a body in-nervated by afferent fibers from one spinal root is a:

A. dermatome
B. myotome
C. sensory distribution pattern
D. peripheral nerve pattern

53. A Trendelenburg gait is an abnormal gait associated with a weakness of which muscle?

A. iliopsoas
B. gluteus maximus
C. gluteus medius
D. tensor fascia lata

54. During the evaluation of a client with a cardiac condition, the client indi-cates the presence of stabbing or burning pain that is made worse by coughing, swallowing, deep breath-ing, and lying down. It is relieved by aspirin and other anti-inflammatory drugs. The pain described is referred to as:

A. pericardial pain
B. pulmonary embolism pain
C. myocardial ischemic pain
D. pain arising from the great vessels

55. During the initial screening of a client referred for pain management, the client reports increased pain and be-comes emotional about no one's be-ing able to help. The pain is de-scribed as constant; lasting all day, every day; and viselike over the ver-tex, yet there are no physical abnor-malities. These findings are consis-tent with:

A. muscle tension
B. organic brain disease
C. conversion hysteria
D. vascular disease

56. A client has an idiopathic "C" curve of more than 60 degrees. Based on the literature, the client will probably have a:

A. decrease in vital capacity
B. higher shoulder on the concave side
C. reluctance to participate in throwing types of sports
D. posterior rib hump on the concave side

57. The _____ originates on the lateral epicondyle of the humerus and the radial collateral lig-ament of the elbow and its covering aponeurosis and inserts on the dor-sal surface of the base of the third metacarpal.

A. extensor digitorum brevis
B. extensor digitorum longus
C. extensor carpi radialis longus
D. extensor carpi radialis brevis

58. If a client has sustained damage to the phrenic nerve, which muscle(s) are expected to be involved?

   A. rectus abdominis
   B. diaphragm
   C. intercostals
   D. lateral obliques

59. The apprehension test has been selected for inclusion in an evaluation. The purpose of this test is to ascertain if:

   A. the patella is dislocating
   B. there is posterior instability of the knee
   C. the menisci are intact
   D. there is anterior instability of the knee

60. The purpose of the Lachman test is to determine if there is:

   A. posterior instability of the knee
   B. anterior instability of the knee
   C. evidence of a patellar lesion
   D. a lateral meniscus tear

61. According to McKenzie, one of the distinguishing features of a derangement syndrome compared with a dysfunction syndrome is:

   A. that they usually occur in women who are 20 to 35 years old
   B. an inability to identify aggravating activities
   C. the presence of intermittent pain
   D. that the person often has constant pain that varies in intensity

62. In the Salter-Harris classification of epiphyseal plate injuries, an intra-articular fracture that extends from the joint surface to the deep zone of the plate and then along the plate to the periphery is what kind of injury?

   A. type I
   B. type II
   C. type III
   D. type IV

63. The anatomical classification of peripheral neuropathies indicates that infections, such as herpes zoster neuronitis, can cause a what kind of neuropathy?

   A. autonomic
   B. somatic sensory
   C. somatic motor
   D. none of the above

64. The most common brain tumors in adults are:

   A. meningiomas
   B. lymphomas
   C. astrocytoma and glioblastoma multiforme
   D. adenomas

65. A child with hydrocephaly will undergo a procedure designed to divert cerebrospinal fluid from the obstructed area of the ventricular system to the subarachnoid space beyond the blockage. This procedure is referred to as:

   A. shunting
   B. bypassing
   C. circumventing
   D. decompressing

66. A client with cardiac disease who experiences slight limitations in physical activity and is comfortable at rest would be described functionally as:

   A. class A
   B. class II
   C. class B
   D. class III

67. A client with cardiac disease whose physical activity does not require restriction is described therapeutically as:

   A. class A
   B. class II
   C. class B
   D. class III

68. **A child's ability to demonstrate fine prehension is being tested. The child is able to hold a thin coin between his thumb and index finger, which is within normal for the client's age. The age of this child is between:**

   A. 1 and 6 months
   B. 7 and 15 months
   C. 5 and 9 months
   D. 2 and 7 months

69. **If a child is able to ambulate alone at 11 months, this would be considered _____ development.**

   A. delayed
   B. early
   C. normal
   D. abnormal

70. **A child who can visually follow past midline but cannot tract 180 degrees or follow objects moved up and down over his or her head would be described as at an age level of:**

   A. 1 to 3 months
   B. 2 to 4 months
   C. 3 to 6 months
   D. 4 to 8 months

71. **The Thomas test is used to assess:**

   A. hamstring tightness
   B. medial instability of the knee
   C. the presence of chondromalacia
   D. hip flexor contractures

72. **A patellar tap test is used to determine:**

   A. ligamentous laxity
   B. significant joint effusion
   C. deep tendon reflexes
   D. sensation and proprioception

73. **According to Cyriax, end feel is the type of resistance felt by an examiner at the:**

   A. end range of a PROM test
   B. beginning range of a PROM test
   C. end range of an AROM test
   D. through range of an AAROM test

74. **Cyriax describes end feel as empty when:**

   A. an abrupt stop occurs in the last 5 degrees of motion after no resistance through the range
   B. there is no resistance throughout the range and excessive motion is possible
   C. the examiner feels no resistance but the client complains of marked pain
   D. there is no bony restriction but the surrounding soft tissues limit the ROM

75. **According to Cyriax, a capsular pattern is a limitation of movement or a pattern of pain at a joint that occurs in a predictable pattern. He believed these patterns are caused by:**

   A. lesions in either the joint capsule or the synovial membrane
   B. surrounding soft tissue damage
   C. habitual abnormal patterns long after an injury has been resolved
   D. inflammation secondary to repetitive stress in a single pattern

76. **According to Kaltenborn's convex-concave rule, when the physical therapist moves a _____ joint surface on a _____ joint surface, the convex joint surface is moved in a direction opposite the ROM limitation.**

   A. concave/convex
   B. convex/convex
   C. concave/concave
   D. convex/concave

77. **When the physical therapist feels resistance at the end range of external rotation of the glenohumeral joint, it is from ligamentous stretching. According to Kaltenborn, this is referred to as a:**

   A. hard end feel
   B. firm end feel
   C. springy end feel
   D. soft end feel

78. **MacConnaill refers to the rotation of a convex joint surface around a longitudinal axis on a concave joint surface as:**

A. slide
B. roll
C. spin
D. glide

79. **Maitland refers to a grade _____ _____ movement when you use small amplitude movements performed at the beginning of the range.**

A. I
B. II
C. III
D. IV

80. **Waddell uses straight-leg raises (SLRs) as a _____ test in diagnosing LBP.**

A. simulation
B. distraction
C. ROM
D. muscle strength

81. **In completing and documenting an evaluation for a client with a diagnosis of rheumatoid arthritis, the functional capacity is documented as class III. This means that the client is:**

A. completely able to perform usual activities of daily living (ADLs)
B. able to perform usual self-care and work-related activities but is limited in avocational activities
C. able to perform usual self-care activities but is limited in both vocational and avocational activities
D. limited in ability to perform usual self-care, vocational, and avocational activities

82. **For the client in item 82 with a diagnosis of rheumatoid arthritis, the stage of progression is documented to be:**

A. stage I, early
B. stage II, moderate
C. stage III, severe
D. stage IV, terminal

83. **A 14-year-old client with a diagnosis of Becker's muscular dystrophy has been referred for evaluation. The client's onset of symptoms began at what age?**

A. 1 to 4 years
B. 5 to 10 years
C. 1 to 10 years
D. 12 to 14 years

84. **Which of the following types of muscular dystrophy is characterized by slow progression with cardiac abnormalities but a normal life span?**

A. Duchenne's
B. Becker's
C. congenital myotonic
D. Emery-Dreifuss

85. **Which of the following types of tests is used to detect potential developmental problems in the areas of gross motor, fine motor, language, and personal-social?**

A. Alberta Infant Motor Scale (AIMS)
B. Chandler Movement Assessment of Infants (CMAI-ST)
C. Denver Development Screening Test II (DDST-II)
D. Early Learning Accomplishment Profile (ELAP)

86. **Which of the following types of tests is used to determine interactive behavior and neuromotor status; state, tone, reflexes, and interactive behavior of a 23-day-old child?**

A. neonatal behavioral assessment scale (NBAS)
B. neonatal oral-motor assessment scale (NOMAS)
C. neurobehavior assessment of preterm infant (NAPI)
D. Milani-Comparetti motor development screening (M-C) Test

87. **Which of the following would be a contraindication for children to participate in competitive contact sports?**

A. mild hypertension
B. atlantoaxial instability
C. well-controlled seizure disorder
D. sickle cell trait

88. After evaluation of a client with end-stage renal disease whose care is paid for by Medicare, treatment is not recommended. The rationale for this recommendation is:

   A. The client does not demonstrate re-habilitation potential.
   B. The client is terminally ill.
   C. The client does not want physical therapy services.
   D. The client's diagnosis is a contraindi-cation for physical therapy interven-tion.

89. The greatest incidence of hip frac-tures in men occurs in what age range?

   A. 50 to 64 years
   B. 65 to 74 years
   C. 75 to 84 years
   D. 85 years and older

90. The leading cause of accidental death in persons 65 years of age is:

   A. automobile collisions
   B. falls
   C. drowning
   D. self-medication

91. An elderly client's home environment is to be assessed before discharge. The major reason for doing so is to assess and offer recommendations regarding:

   A. energy expenditure preservation
   B. adaptive equipment needs
   C. environmental modifications to re-duce the likelihood of falls
   D. the scope of ADLs

92. The test used to assess distant mem-ory in a geriatric client that consists of puzzles or word problems is the:

   A. Extended Dementia Scale
   B. Geriatric Interpersonal Dementia Rat-ing Scale
   C. PGC Mental Status
   D. Wechsler Memory Scale

93. Endogenous depression in the elderly can be tested by using the:

   A. Beck depression inventory
   B. Hopkins symptom checklist
   C. Zung self-rating depression scale
   D. affect balance scale

94. Symptomatic changes that may con-tribute to protein deficiency in older persons include:

   A. chronic depression, fatigue, and ankle fractures
   B. hypertension, hip fractures, and weight loss
   C. loss of social contact, lack of energy, and LBP
   D. reduced muscle strength, pedal edema, and altered thyroid function

95. Which of the following physiological changes may predispose an older in-dividual to hypothermia?

   A. congestive heart failure
   B. arteriosclerosis
   C. compromised proprioception
   D. chronic obstructive lung disease (COPD)

96. After an objective evaluation of a client, a therapist reports what is be-lieved to be causing the client's movement dysfunction. If this belief is not directly supported by evidence, a _____ is being pro-vided.

   A. clinical decision
   B. clinical opinion
   C. dysfunction diagnosis
   D. dysfunction classification

97. The extent to which items that con-tribute to a measurement reflect one basic phenomenon or dimension is the definition of:

   A. internal consistency
   B. inter-tester reliability
   C. intra-tester reliability
   D. parallel forms reliability

98. **Which of the following is a form of validity that deals with the extent to which a measurement is judged to reflect the meaningful elements of a construct and not any extraneous elements?**

   A. construct validity
   B. content validity
   C. criterion-based validity
   D. predictive validity

99. **What is used to determine outcomes for individuals currently participating in rehabilitation programs?**

   A. Fugl-Meyer assessment of sensorimotor recovery after stroke
   B. Functional Independence Measure (FIM)
   C. functional reach test
   D. Gross Motor Performance Measure (GMPM)

100. **The test that is used to determine the functional level of a chronically ill client who is institutionalized is the:**

   A. Motor Assessment Scale (MAS)
   B. Peabody Developmental Motor Scale
   C. PULSES profile
   D. Sorenson test

101. **A client has received the maximum benefit from physical therapy. The administrator of the clinical practice orders the therapist to continue treatment until the client's Medicare coverage maximum is reached. The proper course of action to be taken is to:**

   A. Discharge the client from physical therapy.
   B. Contact the client's primary care physician.
   C. Find some other rehabilitation goal on which to work.
   D. Resign and advise the administrator.

102. **Which one of the following accurately describes the relationship of the thermal effects of ultrasonography?**

   A. increase frequency, decrease heating
   B. decrease protein, increasing heating
   C. decrease blood flow, decrease heating
   D. increase reflection, increase heating

103. **If the intent in applying massage is the reduction of edema, the therapist would:**

   A. Always precede the massage with ice packs.
   B. Begin proximally and proceed distally to proximally.
   C. Use it in conjunction with ultraviolet light therapy.
   D. Follow the massage with superficial heat.

104. **Which one of the following is a contraindication to stretching?**

   A. decreased ROM caused by adhesions
   B. muscle weakness
   C. bony block to joint motion
   D. muscle length imbalance

105. **Autogenic inhibition is:**

   A. a factor that may enhance muscle stretching
   B. a precaution in muscle stretching of aging clients
   C. a method of inhibiting the tight muscle by eliciting a contraction of its antagonist muscle
   D. present in clients with neurological dysfunctions whose muscles have been overstretched

106. **The most accurate description of the technique of timing for emphasis is:**

   A. giving a quick stretch at the beginning of the pattern
   B. passively moving the limb through the pattern
   C. holding back all but one of the components of the pattern
   D. resisting patterns in positions other than supine

107. **For a client who lacks eccentric control of scapular posterior elevation musculature, which of the following proprioceptive neuromuscular facilitation (PNF) patterns would best address his problem?**

A. resisted upper extremity (UE) D2 extension pattern with tubing attached at client's foot
B. resisted UE D1 flexion pattern with tubing attached at client's foot
C. resisted UE D2 flexion pattern with tubing attached above client's head
D. resisted UE D1 extension pattern with tubing attached above client's head

108. **A 36-year-old construction worker who sustained a lumbar injury is enrolled in a work-hardening program. All of the following are typical components of a program except:**

A. work simulation
B. body mechanics education
C. management of symptoms of pain
D. functional capacity evaluation and reevaluation

109. **Which one of the following statements is an example of the relaxation technique of neuromuscular dissociation?**

A. "Tense your right biceps while keeping all of the rest of your muscles relaxed."
B. "See yourself lying on a warm sunny beach. As each wave rolls out to the sea, you slowly let go of the tension in your forearm."
C. "As I touch your right biceps, let the tension melt and roll out of your arm."
D. "Repeat to yourself 'My arm is heavy. My arm is warm. My arm is completely relaxed.' Repeat this process for 3 to 5 minutes each day."

110. **A 45-year-old, 180-lb client complains of LBP with radiating pain down the back of left leg to the ankle. Pain has been present for 12 days. During the initial visit, lumbar static traction was included as part of the treatment. The traction was applied in the supine position for 10 minutes at 90 lbs. It is now 2 days later, and the client's symptoms increased after the last visit. In light of this subjective information, which of the following is most appropriate?**

A. increase the poundage to 100 lbs
B. increase the time of the treatment to 20 minutes
C. decrease the poundage of traction
D decrease the length of time of the treatment to 5 minutes

111. **The client is a 46-year-old public health nurse who carried a heavy portable electrocardiographic machine on the right shoulder to and from the car 2 weeks ago. The client was awakened that night by severe LBP, right leg pain, and numbness in the right foot. The client has not gone to work for 2 weeks. Pain has decreased in intensity with decreased activity; however, LBP, right lower extremity (RLE) pain and right foot numbness persist. There is no other history of injury. Bilateral SLRs elicit LBP as the lumbar spine moves. In standing, posture reflects bilateral hip and knee flexion, hip adduction, and genu valgum. Movements are still guarded and tentative. The lumbopelvic region is still tender to bilateral palpation. The client reports a decrease in pain with grade II manual traction but complains of increased pain with grade III. Based on this information, today it is appropriate to apply:**

A. manual traction without tissue stretch
B. manual traction with tissue stretch short of end range
C. manual traction with tissue stretch to end of physiological range
D. mechanical traction to one half of body weight

112. For the client in item 111, instruction in correct sitting posture was also included in the treatment plan. The client was advised **not** to engage in:

A. reclined sitting
B. erect sitting
C. slump sitting
D. forward sitting

113. While using a PNF pattern, manual contact is applied to resist the anterior elevation pattern of the pelvis. The resistance is limited to the:

A. iliac crest just above the ASIS
B. level of the ASIS
C. ischial tuberosity
D. trochanter of the femur

114. When considering client movement during a gait training session, the pelvic pattern during the midswing phase of gait on the swing leg side is most accurately described as:

A. posterior depression
B. anterior elevation
C. posterior elevation
D. anterior depression

115. The client was referred for management of LBP secondary to a strain of the iliolumbar ligament. He has a subacute status but continues to move very stiffly because of excessive muscle splinting. Maximum pain level is 5 on a scale of 10. The most appropriate initial technique while working with PNF pelvic patterns would be:

A. slow reversals to improve active movement
B. rhythmic initiation to encourage muscle relaxation
C. combined isotonics to encourage muscle relaxation
D. passive movement only

116. In the middle of a treatment session, a 13-year-old client with a diagnosis of T-12 level paraplegia begins to talk about the automobile accident that led to his disability. Because the other occupants of the car were killed, little information has been available. For the first time, it is acknowledged that a passenger was a gang member and that the car was deliberately run off the road on a hillside by members of a rival gang. Before this conversation, it was difficult to get the client to learn and perform strengthening exercises, transfer training, and ADLs. According to Maslow's hierarchy of needs, the client may be experiencing difficulty in learning because his or her
_____ needs have not been met.

A. self-actualization
B. love and respect
C. safety and survival
D. self-esteem

117. When teaching a client who has undergone a total hip replacement to perform a functional activity, such as transferring from sitting to standing, the primary goal or objective should be within which domain (according to Bloom)?

A. cognitive
B. integrative
C. affective
D. psychomotor

118. As the supervising therapist for inpatient services in a skilled nursing facility (SNF), one of the staff therapists was observed shouting at a client and repeating commands rapidly. The client appeared to be becoming confused and less able to perform her exercise program. The therapist is advised to give the client time to practice without continuous feedback and that his tone of voice needs to be calmer and quieter. The rationale for this position is:

A. There is a difference between performance and learning.
B. Timing of feedback is critical for learning to occur.
C. The client is emotionally upset with the therapy session.
D. The therapist seems to be acting condescendingly toward the client.

119. A client asks what level of education the physical therapist assistant in the department has. The appropriate reply is that the educational requirements specified in your state law require graduation from an accredited education program. The accreditation criteria specify that the assistant must possess a/an:

A. associate's degree
B. baccalaureate degree
C. certification of completion
D. high school diploma and completion of a vocational technical program

120. The client in item 119 then asks if the treating therapist has a license. The response is that the therapist recently graduated from a master of physical therapy (MPT) degree program, took the examination 2 weeks ago, and that by law is considered to:

A. be a registered physical therapist
B. have a temporary license
C. be a license applicant
D. be a licensed physical therapist

121. In most states, physical therapists are permitted to evaluate and treat clients without a referral from a physician. This is commonly referred to as:

A. autonomy
B. direct access
C. independent practice
D. professional status

122. The method of payment for the services a client receives has an established maximum dollar amount for services provided. This method of payment is commonly referred to as:

A. capitation
B. rationing
C. fee for service
D. indemnification

123. When a provider of care is forced to make a decision that violates one of the principles of medical ethics in order to adhere to another principle, the situation is referred to as a/an:

A. moral conflict
B. ethical issue
C. maleficence
D. ethical dilemma

124. A colleague has been documenting treatments that were not given. The ethical and legal obligation for any therapist with direct knowledge is to:

A. Confront the colleague about his behavior and report it to the facility administrator.
B. Report the therapist to the licensing agency.
C. Request termination of employment of the offending therapist.
D. Report the overcharges to the clients' payors.

125. **When applying electrical stimulation, knowledge of motor points is essential. These are sites:**

   A. on the skin surface where the underlying muscle can be electrically stimulated
   B. directly over the underlying muscle belly
   C. that correspond to the acupuncture points for needle insertion
   D. for placement of surface electrodes for electroneuromyographic testing

126. **When a muscle contracts in response to stimulation with galvanic (direct) current but not in response to faradic (alternating) current, the phenomenon is referred to as:**

   A. denervation
   B. rheobase response
   C. reaction to degeneration
   D. regeneration

127. **When interferential current is applied, the waveform is/are:**

   A. twin peak pulses
   B. continuous sine wave
   C. direct
   D. sine wave

128. **In administering low-voltage electrical stimulation, the intensity is:**

   A. less than 150 volts
   B. 90 to 100 mA
   C. 150 to 175 volts
   D. 70 to 90 mA

129. **A client is just beginning to have return of movement within a flexor synergy pattern in her UE. Brunnstrom techniques are being used with this client. At this stage it is appropriate to use:**

   A. scapular techniques to facilitate elevation and retraction because these are often the first motions to return within the synergy pattern
   B. rowing in and out of flexor synergy, emphasizing the movement out of synergy in order to facilitate normal movement patterns
   C. finger extension techniques (rolling, swatting, molding) to facilitate finger extension because normal movement patterns return in distal areas before proximal areas
   D. any of the above three techniques are appropriate for this client at this stage of recovery

130. **A progression of PNF techniques based on developmental strategies to improve motor control is:**

   A. rhythmic stabilization, slow reversals, rhythmic initiation, repeated contraction
   B. prone on elbows, one-leg stance, quadruped, kneeling
   C. rhythmic initiation, rhythmic stabilization, slow reversals
   D. sidelying, supine, long sitting, prone, quadruped

131. **A different therapist is taking over the management of a client with an SCI. Which of the following is not true regarding management of secondary complications of SCI?**

   A. Examine the skin for redness and do periodic pressure relief techniques.
   B. During autonomic dysreflexia, remove restrictive clothing and have the client lie down.
   C. Use stretching to combat heterotopic bone formation.
   D. Use abdominal binders and long support stockings to prevent orthostatic hypotension.

132. **Yesterday an 82-year-old client was evaluated for residual deficits secondary to a CVA. The three primary problems with which the therapist is working include decreased balance, decreased AROM LLE, and dependence in all functional activities. The appropriate choice of techniques and position to use for strengthening trunk extensors are:**

A. Brunnstrom: forward flexion with arms cradled, semi-sitting
B. PNF: approximation through the shoulders, adding resistance in sitting
C. rowing in synergy with resistance only in extension
D. neurodevelopmental techniques (NDTs): align and then facilitate standing weight shift in diagonals

133. **For the client in item 132, it is now 2 weeks later, and work continues on trunk extension. Which of the following is the most appropriate technique and positioning?**

A. Brunnstrom: assisted forward flexion with arms cradled, sitting
B. PNF: chopping pattern in supine
C. Swiss ball-sitting activities
D. both A and C because they would facilitate greater gain

134. **A new client is being seen today in the intensive care unit. The client is 21 years old and suffered a closed head injury. A chest tube is in place. Sensory stimulation has been chosen as an intervention. All of the following are true except:**

A. An appropriate auditory stimulation would be to leave the radio or TV on for background sounds.
B. Motor responses, such as eye movements, facial grimacing, changes in posture, head turning, or vocalization, should be documented.
C. Sensory stimulation is theorized to activate the reticular activating system, causing a general increase in arousal.
D. Vestibular stimulation can be provided by neck ROM, rolling on the bed, rocking, or pushing the client in a wheelchair.

135. **A 14-year-old client sustained a head injury when a drunk driver struck him while he was riding a bicycle. According to the Rancho Los Amigos stage of cognitive function, if the client appears oriented to place but performs ADLs in a robot-like way and requires at least minimal supervision for safety, the cognitive level is:**

A. stage III, localized response
B. stage VII, automatic and appropriate
C. stage VIII, unsafe, appropriate
D. stage IV, purposeful, oriented

136. **Three of four clients seen today demonstrated visual or perceptual disturbances. This was consistent with the literature, which indicates these disturbances are common in individuals with these diagnoses. Clients with which disorders did not experience visual or perceptual disturbances?**

A. SCI
B. CVA
C. TIA
D. multiple sclerosis

137. **A 2-year-old child undergoing treatment has had a sacrococcygeal teratoma surgically removed. As the therapist works with the child to resume ambulation, the mother asks what her child's prognosis is. The legal and ethical response is:**

   A. "I can't answer that for you. Only your physician can discuss this with you."
   B. "Have you spoken with your physician about her future? Most of these tumors are benign."
   C. "I don't really know and can't answer your question."
   D. "There are several books in the medical library that you might want to check out so you will know for yourself."

138. **The members of the primary care team for clients with SCIs are discussing weaning a client from a ventilator. Which ventilator mode would immediately precede progression to continuous positive airway pressure (CPAP)?**

   A. synchronized intermittent mandatory ventilation (SIMV)
   B. assist control
   C. control
   D. assist

139. **Which of the following is not a contraindication to percussion during postural drainage?**

   A. rib fracture
   B. hemothorax
   C. sonorous rhonchi
   D. empyema

140. **Gait training with axillary crutches has been delegated to a physical therapist assistant with instructions to use a three-point non–weight-bearing pattern. The client has a medical diagnosis of a fracture of the right tibia. The rationale for delegating this treatment is that:**

   A. The assistant has been working with the therapist for more than 1 year and appears to be confident and competent.
   B. The roles and functions of the therapist in the managed-care environment are primarily that of evaluation and diagnosis.
   C. The administrator has advised that routine care must be delegated to the supportive personnel in the department.
   D. It is within the scope of practice of the physical therapist assistant.

141. **A client with a diagnosis of COPD has been in the hospital for 3 days and is now ready for discharge. Physical therapy is requested for a predischarge assessment. The interview reveals that the client lives alone but a neighbor helps with meals. The client ambulated short distances independently before admission and has no stairs into or in the house. SaO_2 level at rest on 2 L of oxygen by nasal cannula is 97%. During the treatment session, the client ambulates slowly on room air for 50 feet independently, is mildly short of breath, and fatigues after walking. SaO_2 level on room air after ambulation is 92%. Which of the following would be the best plan for this client's discharge from the hospital?**

   A. Discharge home with supplemental oxygen and instructions on energy conservation techniques.
   B. Discharge home without supplemental oxygen and instructions on energy conservation techniques.
   C. SNF for physical therapy with supplemental oxygen and instructions on energy conservation techniques.
   D. Bedrest with instructions on energy conservation techniques and the requirement of a live-in home care aide.

142. **Three reflexes have been identified as potentially affecting the diameter of the thoracic outlet and the blood flow to the UE. The most common and most frequently overlooked dysfunctional reflex is:**

   A. a paradoxical breathing pattern
   B. the flexion withdrawal reflex
   C. vasoconstriction
   D. vasodilatation

143. **After evaluation, it is determined that a client has an anteriorly rotated right ilium that contributes to pain symptoms. Which of the following are appropriate in a home program?**

   A. isometric contractions of right hip flexors and left hip extensors
   B. use the gluteus minimus by positioning the left hip in 90 degrees flexion with abduction and external rotation and resisting adduction
   C. isometric contractions of the left hip flexors and the right hip extensors
   D. isotonic trunk rotation to the right

144. **An exercise program is designed to strengthen the musculature for depression of the humerus on the glenoid. This exercise is primarily for which muscle?**

   A. pectoralis major
   B. pectoralis minor
   C. subclavius
   D. supraspinatus

145. **A client has limited UE elevation. The physical therapist's evaluation revealed limited clavicular elevation. The plan of care includes mobilization of the sternoclavicular joint. Which of the following accessory movements would be appropriate to accomplish this task?**

   A. anterior to posterior
   B. posterior to anterior
   C. rostral to caudal
   D. caudal to rostral

146. **Stretching exercises of the _____ _____ have been included in an exercise program in order to reduce a lumbar flexion restriction.**

   A. erector spinae and hamstrings
   B. hamstrings and psoas
   C. psoas and erector spinae
   D. psoas and gluteals

147. **During treatment of a 48-year-old writer with a musculoskeletal dysfunction involving the scapular musculature, a technique is used in which the client is asked to attempt to find the point on his back where the therapist's finger is and allow the tightness to "melt like butter." This is an example of:**

   A. superficial myofascial release
   B. deep myofascial release
   C. craniosacral alignment
   D. creative visualization

148. **In a strengthening exercise program involving manual resistance and forceful adduction of the arm, the pull of the teres major on the scapula is stabilized by the:**

   A. serratus anterior
   B. rhomboids
   C. deltoid
   D. trapezius

149. **A client is working on an exercise program to decrease tight hamstrings. The client's gait before initiation of the program was characterized by:**

   A. shortened stride length
   B. lumbar spine flexion
   C. posterior pelvic tilt
   D. all of the above

150. A client who underwent arthroscopic removal of a torn medial meniscus was instructed to perform standing quadriceps exercises. The client's performance is observed, and it is concluded that there is normal biomechanical motion at the knee. The movement at the knee would therefore be the:

A. femur rolls forward and then glides back
B. femur rolls back and then glides forward
C. tibia rolls forward and then glides back
D. tibia rolls back and then glides forward

151. Intervention is directed at bilaterally lengthening the suboccipital muscles. However, the client has compensated for this shortening by:

A. cervical side bending
B. flexing at the lower cervical spine
C. opening the jaw
D. extending the lumbar spine

152. A client demonstrates weak upper limb abduction but normal ROM and weak and limited active flexion (0 to 130 degrees) with normal passive range. The exercise program will be targeted to increase the strength of the:

A. trapezius
B. deltoid
C. serratus anterior
D. pectoralis major

153. An exercise program involves having the peroneus longus and tibialis posterior function as a force couple. Which motion will the client be performing?

A. plantarflexion
B. inversion
C. dorsiflexion
D. eversion

154. A client has been receiving physical therapy to increase gastrocnemius/soleus muscle strength. The muscle weakness is accompanied by numbness and tingling in the foot with no symptoms in the thigh or posterior calf. This would likely be a result of:

A. peroneal nerve compression as it winds around the lateral malleolus
B. tibial nerve compression in the tarsal tunnel
C. compression of lateral plantar nerve in the heel region
D. compression of medial plantar nerve in the heel region

155. A client has a movement dysfunction that includes limited ability to extend the knee and flex the thigh. The client's history includes a back strain injury just before the emergence of the weakness in the lower extremity (LE). Treatment today will include posterior-to-anterior mobilization of:

A. T-12
B. L3
C. L5
D. S-1/2

156. If a client's treatment program is designed to increase strength in order to perform functional activities involving lateral or external rotation of the shoulder, resistive exercises will be used primarily for the:

A. infraspinatus
B. deltoid
C. latissimus dorsi
D. supraspinatus

157. A home exercise pool program designed to foster increased endurance should include:

A. walking laps for 5 to 10 minutes
B. UE weightlifting in the pool
C. stretching exercises of the hip flexors and knee extensors
D. the crawl and breast strokes for multiple laps

158. **Starting at the anterior superior iliac spine and moving laterally along the iliac crest, which muscle can be palpated?**

   A. sartorius
   B. rectus femoris
   C. gluteus medius
   D. tensor fascia lata

159. **In distal segment fixed activities, right hip internal rotation is paired with lumbar spine:**

   A. extension
   B. flexion
   C. rotation left
   D. rotation right

160. **Of the following definitions, which best describes skeletal muscle?**

   A. multinucleated, striated, and cylindrical
   B. single nucleus, striated, and branched
   C. multinucleated, striated, and fusiform
   D. single nucleus, unstriated, and fusiform

161. **The client is a 45-year-old woman who underwent a left mastectomy followed by reconstruction using the TRAM procedure. In the first treatment session since the TRAM procedure, the most appropriate treatment to provide is:**

   A. AAROM and AROM of the LUE to facilitate full ROM
   B. bilateral UE strengthening exercises and edema-reduction positioning
   C. ADLs with minimal assistance for bed mobility
   D. instruction in proper body mechanics to reduce stress on the sutures

162. **A client is placed in a sidelying position and instructed to flex the hip to 90 degrees. That motion occurs around the _____ axis in the _____ plane.**

   A. anteroposterior/frontal
   B. frontal/sagittal
   C. longitudinal/transverse
   D. horizontal/coronal

163. **As the rate of loading increases, the stiffness of both bone and cartilage:**

   A. increases
   B. decreases
   C. does not change
   D. decreases and then increases

164. **In documenting the progress that a client made during today's treatment session, you should emphasize the:**

   A. level of strength, ROM, and endurance
   B. short-term goal achievement expressed in functional outcomes
   C. ADL improvements since yesterday
   D. potential for accomplishing long-term goals

165. **In cases of acute locked spinal joints, manually delivered passive joint movements (MPMs) often result in immediate relief of severe pain. The assumption is that:**

   A. MPM moves or frees the impediment, permitting movement and halting nociceptive input and associated reflex muscle spasm.
   B. The patient is distracted from focusing on the pain and thus the central nervous system (CNS) can accommodate to the pain.
   C. MPM decreases joint irritability by facilitating normal movement.
   D. The procedure is comfortable to the client and relaxation will help the impediment to dislodge itself.

166. **A research project that involves the use of control groups and randomization is referred to as:**

   A. descriptive
   B. experimental
   C. phenomenological
   D. quasi-experimental

167. In a research project, when the numbers or symbols assigned to objects have no numerical meaning beyond the presence or absence of an attribute being measured, the measurement is referred to as:

A. ordinal
B. nominal
C. encoded
D. inferential

168. Chi-square data are commonly referred to as _____ statistics.

A. parametric
B. nonparametric
C. means comparison
D. correlation

169. In measuring the differences between group means, the most commonly used test is the:

A. *t* test
B. chi-square test
C. Wilcoxon test
D. Mann Whitney test

170. In a research project in your department, the analysis of data will include more than one dependent variable. The test most commonly used in this situation is the:

A. Wilcoxon sign
B. multivariate analysis of variance (MANOVA)
C. analysis of variance (ANOVA)
D. Mann Whitney test

171. In a client with acquired immunodeficiency syndrome, visual deficits are often caused by:

A. *Mycobacterium avium intracellulare*
B. tuberculosis
C. *Cytomegalovirus*
D. thrush

172. An individual with a diagnosis of metastatic cancer undergoing chemotherapy may exhibit a decrease in platelet counts. This is referred to as:

A. leukopenia
B. anemia
C. thrombocytopenia
D. pancytopenia

173. A client recently underwent colon surgery secondary to a new diagnosis of colon cancer. It is 1 week after surgery and the client is taking tube feedings and is resuming physical therapy. In which phase within the rehabilitation continuum is this client?

A. palliative
B. restorative
C. supportive
D. communicative

174. In the case of a full-thickness burn, it would be consistent to see:

A. variable sensation in the wound bed
B. rapid re-epithelialization from dermal elements
C. re-epithelialization from wound edges only
D. risk of bacterial conversion

175. A nonblanchable erythema of the skin is referred to as:

A. hypertrophic scar tissue
B. grade I ulceration
C. toxic epidermal necrolysis
D. zone of stasis

176. Ultrasonography has been included in a care plan for a client with a nonhealing wound. The rationale is that ultrasonography will:

A. Increase collagen synthesis and improve tensile strength of tissue.
B. Destroy *Staphylococcus aureus* bacteria.
C. Increase capillary bed formation.
D. Decrease pain.

177. **Attempting to foster a sense of self and accomplishment in a client is an attempt to foster:**

A. sympathy
B. empowerment
C. interchangeable empathy
D. behavior modification

178. **The requirement to contact a payor before the provision of physical therapy services is:**

A. a common requirement for therapists whose claims have been investigated
B. to guarantee the client that appropriate services will be provided
C. prior authorization
D. capitation

179. **Research studies have shown that the maximum penetration of topical agents via phonophoresis is:**

A. < 0.5 inch
B. > 0.5 inch
C. < 5.0 cm
D. > 5.0 cm

180. **Outriggers on an UE orthosis are designed to:**

A. facilitate flexor strengthening
B. increase ROM
C. maintain and permit extension ROM
D. approximate normal wrist and hand positioning

181. **The most appropriate assistive device for gait training of a 35-year-old client who is a low–level (L4/5) paraplegic is/are:**

A. a standard walker
B. bilateral quadriped canes
C. axillary crutches
D. forearm crutches

182. **One of the major social problems encountered by persons with a medical diagnosis of cancer is:**

A. community rejection
B. feelings of helplessness and hopelessness
C. lower socioeconomic status
D. societally limited resources

183. **Physical therapists in hospice programs assist clients in:**

A. areas of mobility
B. endurance development
C. strengthening
D. gait training

184. **A 15-year-old client recently underwent an above-the-knee amputation secondary to a diagnosis of bone cancer. The client is being seen 4 days after the amputation. The program to be implemented today is most likely:**

A. residual limb conditioning
B. bed mobility and transfer training
C. gait training
D. all of the above

185. **The heart is innervated by both the sympathetic and parasympathetic nervous systems. Sympathetic nervous system (SNS) efferent fibers originate in the _____ _____ region; proceed through the superior, middle, and inferior cervical ganglia; and end in the atria and ventricles.**

A. cervicothoracic
B. thoracolumbar
C. upper thoracic
D. lumbosacral

186. **The primary neurotransmitter for the parasympathetic nervous system is:**

A. acetylcholine
B. epinephrine
C. norepinephrine
D. dopamine

187. **A client with chronic heart failure has received physical therapy for 2 weeks. The care plan is focused on inspiratory muscle training. Which of the following is consistent with current research findings?**

A. There are no changes in maximal inspiratory pressure (MIP) and dyspnea.
B. There are improvements in MIP, maximal expiratory pressure (MEP), and dyspnea.
C. There is improvement in MIP but no change in MEP.
D. There is improvement in MIP and MEP but no change in dyspnea.

188. **Of the following procedures, which has been used for edema reduction in clients with lymphedema?**

A. cryotherapy
B. phonophoresis
C. whirlpool and Hubbard tank
D. iontophoresis

189. **Conduction velocity is defined as:**

A. an electrochemical event associated with the propagation of a wave of depolarization along the length of an excitable cell
B. the transmission of nerve impulses over motor nerves away from the CNS
C. the speed with which a volley of nerve impulses travels along a bundle of nerve fibers
D. the speed of transmission of nerve impulses over sensory nerves toward the CNS

190. **The most common use for transcutaneous electrical nerve stimulation (TENS) is:**

A. postsurgical pain
B. chronic LBP
C. pain related to bone cancers
D. acute LBP

191. **Enkephalins, endorphins, serotonin, and dopamine operate in different parts of the CNS and are collectively referred to as:**

A. endogenous opiates
B. healing hormones
C. chemicals released by the substantia gelatinosa
D. somatosensory signals

192. **A client presents with symptoms characteristic of a posterior bulging disk at L-3. An appropriate initial exercise program will focus on:**

A. lateral trunk flexion
B. posterior pelvic tilt
C. lumbar extension
D. left thoracolumbar rotation

193. **A major branch of the cervical plexus that innervates the diaphragm is the**

_____ nerve.

A. accessory
B. thoracodorsal
C. vagus
D. phrenic

194. **When documenting functional outcomes, it is essential that they be:**

A. short term
B. measurable
C. in concert with the client's insurance
D. comprehensive

195. **Administration of intermittent compression to a client with UE edema has been delegated to an experienced physical therapist assistant. The parameters for UE and LE treatments have been established. Which of the following is appropriate for a client who demonstrates edema of the UE?**

A. 20 to 5 0 mm Hg
B. 30 to 70 mm Hg
C. 40 to 80 mm Hg
D. 50 to 90 mm Hg

196. **A client is 56 years old and has diabetes and coronary artery disease. The goal of your aerobic exercise program at this point in time is to:**

A. improve the client's functional ability level.
B. modify the risk factor of glucose intolerance.
C. condition the client overall before bypass surgery.
D. improve the client's self-image.

197. **The most common pulmonary emboli occur after:**

A. coronary artery bypass surgery
B. infectious pneumonia
C. deep vein thrombosis in the LE
D. a period of repeated asthma attacks

198. **The therapeutic objective of a diaphragmatic breathing exercise program is to:**

A. Improve oxygenation and ventilation.
B. Decrease client dependence and depression.
C. Alleviate dyspnea and improve the ease of breathing.
D. Decrease the respiratory rate.

199. **In working with a client who is on bedrest for phlebitis, you decide that your ADL program will begin with:**

A. rolling side to side at least every 2 hours
B. UE strengthening and LE AROM exercises
C. long sitting general mobility exercises for the UEs
D. reciprocal UE and LE AROM exercises

200. **One of the serious side effects of mechanical ventilation is:**

A. increased risk of pulmonary infection
B. inability to communicate
C. psychological dependency
D. inability to perform ADLs

Selecting a Bibliography

There are thousands of articles and books that are relevant to physical therapy. You can spend a fortune in both time and money attempting to read as much of the literature as possible. Instead, it is recommended that you determine the areas in which you need to improve your knowledge and competence and then do a literature search on the Internet or in a college or university library database to identify the most current literature. If you have access to the Internet, you will be able to secure an annotated bibliography and possibly copies of the articles themselves. You should use a medical library for the majority of references. Call ahead to ascertain if the journals that you are seeking are available. You will find that the reference librarians are very helpful.

Generally, the practice is to look at articles and texts that are no more than 10 years old unless, of course, they are considered to be the classics in the profession. The following references are offered as examples of contemporary research within physical therapy and medicine in the past decade that have led us to practice differently. This is merely a sampling.

Bangart, S: Managed care contract checklist. PT Mag of Phys Ther 1993, Jul:26–28.

Benson, HA, and McElnay, JC: Topical NSAID products as ultrasound couplants: Their potential in phonophoresis. Physiotherapy 1994, 80:74.

Bogduk, N, and Twomey, L: Clinical Anatomy of the Lumbar Spine. New York, Churchill Livingstone, 1987.

Butler, D: Mobilization of the Nervous System. New York, Churchill Livingstone, 1991.

Cyriax, J: Textbook of Orthopaedic Medicine, vols I and 2. Baltimore, Williams & Wilkins, 1986. (This is a classic and is therefore included.)

Derosa, CP, and Porterfield, JA: A physical therapy model for the treatment of low back pain. Phys Ther 1992, 72:261–268.

Dougherty, C: Ethical principles in health care reform. PT Mag of Phys Ther 1993, Dec:58–59.

Emwemeka, CS: Laser biostimulation of healing wounds: Specific effects and mechanisms of action. J Ortho Sport Phys Ther 1988, 9:333–338.

Grant, R: Physical Therapy of the Cervical and Thoracic Spine. New York, Churchill Livingstone, 1994.

Grieve, G: Modern Manual Therapy of the Vertebral Column. New York, Churchill Livingstone, 1986. (This is now considered a classic in manual therapy.)

Grieve, G: Common Vertebral Joint Problems. New York, Churchill Livingstone, 1981. (This is now considered a classic in manual therapy.)

Kitchen and Partridge: A review of therapeutic ultrasound. Physiology 1990, 76:593–600.

Monahan, B: Managing under managed care. PT Mag of Phys Ther 1994, Jul:34–40.

Nussbaum, EL, Biemann, I, and Mustard, B: Comparison of ultrasound/ultraviolet–C and laser for treatment of pressure ulcers in patients with spinal cord injury. Phys Ther 1994, 74:812.

Portney, L, and Watkins, M. Foundations of Clinical Research: Applications to Practice. East Norwalk, CT, Appleton & Lange, 1993.

Purtilo, R: To move beyond private opinion. PT Mag of Phys Ther 1993, Jan: 94–100.

Purtilo, R: An instrument of our own minds. PT Mag of Phys Ther 1993, Feb:76–78.

Sicard-Rosenbaum, L, Lord, D, Danoff, JV, et al.: Effects of continuous therapeutic ultrasound on growth and metastasis of subcutaneous murine tumors. Phys Ther 1995, 75:3.

Shamberger, RC, et al.: The effect of ultrasonic and thermal treatment on wounds. Plast Reconstr Surg 1981, 68:860. (This is a classic article.)

Twomey, L, and Taylor, J (eds): Physical Therapy of the Low Back. New York, Churchill Livingstone, 1994.

The references included in each of the chapters of this book represent the most commonly used texts and associated articles. They are certainly not inclusive of all of the references you could read. However, you may find them helpful as you attempt to focus your studying for the examination.

Correct Answers to Comprehensive Multiple Choice Examination

1. B	51. A	101. A	151. B
2. A	52. A	102. D	152. C
3. D	53. C	103. B	153. B
4. B	54. A	104. C	154. B
5. A	55. C	105. A	155. C
6. 6	56. A	106. C	156. D
7 C	57. C	107. B	157. A
8. C	58. B	108. C	158. D
9. A	59. A	109. A	159. C
10. C	60. B	110. C	160. A
11. B	61. D	111. B	161. D
12. C	62. C	112. D	162. B
13. B	63. B	113. A	163. A
14. D	64. C	114. B	164. B
15. B	65. A	115. B	165. A
16. A	66. D	116. C	166. D
17. C	67. A	117. D	167. B
18. A	68. B	118. B	168. B
19. D	69. C	119. A	169. A
20. C	70. A	120. C	170. B
21. B	71. D	121. B	171. C
22. D	72. B	122. A	172. C
23. B	73. A	123. D	173. B
24. A	74. C	124. B	174. C
25. C	75. A	125. A	175. B
26. D	76. D	126. C	176. C
27. B	77. B	127. D	177. B
28. D	78. C	128. A	178. C
29. B	79. A	129. A	179. A
30. C	80. B	130. C	180. C
31. A	81. C	131. B	181. D
32. C	82. B	132. B	182. C
33. B	83. B	133. C	183. A
34. A	84. D	134. A	184. D
35. B	85. C	135. B	185. B
36. C	86. A	136. A	186. A
37. A	87. B	137. B	187. B
38. B	88. A	138. A	188. D
39. D	89. D	139. C	189. C
40. A	90. B	140. D	190. B
41. B	91. C	141. B	191. A
42. D	92. B	142. A	192. C
43. A	93. A	143. C	193. D
44. D	94. D	144. A	194. B
45. C	95. C	145. D	195. A
46. A	96. B	146. C	196. B
47. C	97. A	147. A	197. C
48. B	98. B	148. B	198. C
49. A	99. B	149. D	199. A
50. B	100. C	150. A	200. A